R.J. STEWART

THE MYSTIC LIFE OF MERLIN

R.J. Stewart is a Scot, a musician, composer and author. He has written books and essays on music, folklore, mythology and symbolism, and has a long-standing involvement with Western esoteric traditions. He has composed for feature films, television, radio and stage, and has recorded a number of LP records, tuitional and meditational tapes.

R.J. STEWART

THE MYSTIC LIFE OF MERLIN

WITH ORIGINAL ILLUSTRATIONS BY FELICITY BOWERS

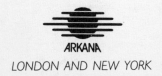

ARKANA

LONDON AND NEW YORK

First published in 1986
Reprinted in 1987 by
Routledge & Kegan Paul Ltd
11 New Fetter Lane, London EC4P 4EE

Published in the USA by
Routledge & Kegan Paul Inc.
in association with Methuen Inc.
29 West 35th Street, New York, NY 10001

Set in Sabon 10/11½pt.
by Columns of Reading
and printed in Great Britain
by The Guernsey Press Co Ltd
Guernsey, Channel Islands

Library of Congress Cataloging in Publication Data
Stewart, R. J., 1949-
The mystic life of Merlin.
Contains an English translation of Geoffey of
Monmouth's Vita Merlini.
Bibliography: p.
Includes index.
1. Geoffrey, of Monmouth, Bishop of St. Asaph,
1100?-1154. Vita Merlini.   2. Merlin — Legends —
History and criticism.   3. Merlin — Legends.
I. Geoffrey, of Monmouth, Bishop of St. Asaph, 1100?-
1154. Vita Merlini.   English. 1986.   II. Title.
PA8310.G4A737   1986   873'.03   86-10876

British Library CIP Data also available
ISBN 1-85063-042-9

Contents

Illustrations

Preface and reader's guide

All these things shall Three Ages see, till the buried Kings shall be exposed to public view in the city of London.

Prophecies of Merlin

The aims of this book are specific and deliberately limited; to reveal certain internal symbolic structures and methods of transpersonal growth found within the twelfth-century *Vita Merlini, The Life of Merlin*. Here is magic, psychology, myth and legend, and some enduring spiritual or timeless wisdom. It would be hard to find even the most obdurate materialist who cannot identify with one of the interwoven themes in the original plot, for it consists of pairs of opposing and complementary world-views ranging from the style and merits of the great worldly leader to the inspirational fits of the wild man of the woods; from the sensual beauty of the natural female to the intellectual and progressive development of a very emancipated and intelligent woman who controls much of the action with or without the consent or knowledge of the men around her.

These polarised and mutually balancing characters react upon one another through the central figure of Merlin, who ultimately achieves an awareness that is utterly transformed by his adventures. On our long and spiralling path through these adventures, the original author has set out vast diversions and complex interweavings of information, cultural lore and heritage, poetry, cosmology, geography, invocation, psychic analysis, magical tuition, and a great deal of hidden symbolism that lies barely below the surface of the rational narrative text. It is this last area which I have specifically tried to expose to public view, rather like the buried kings in Westminster whose exhibition was accurately predicted by Merlin in his *Prophecies* so many centuries past.

The foundation of the *Vita* is a combination of classical or post-classical knowledge available to the medieval scholar, fused in a curious and quite cunning manner with British Celtic legends. The legendary element and the classical derivations both contain psychological and magical symbols of enduring value; the application of such symbols changes from century to century and person to person but their broad basis as keys to the imaginative consciousness remains firm.

As the *Vita* is long and publishing space is short, I have intentionally limited this study to the major patterns and symbols which seem directly valuable and interesting to the modern reader; particularly those which are of Celtic or Western origin, but not exclusively so. No claim is made that this is a complete or fully definitive analysis; it is an essay towards the roots of such an analysis for the general reader, and not a true academic or critical book in the scholarly sense. At this stage it is worth listing briefly the various deliberate omissions, and the fact that many of these areas are dealt with in other books at great length.

I have excluded many literary and linguistic matters, which are found in the various reference books cited; most derivative material from classical sources which carry an enormous weight of modern literature in their own right; and most of the prophetic political verses from the *Vita*, which are found in the translations. There is very little apocalyptic vision in the *Vita*, so there is no need for repetition of the theories on prophetic symbolism outlined in my previous book *The Prophetic Vision of Merlin*, which dealt with the bizarre but by no means incomprehensible text that predates the *Vita* by several years. To grasp some of the principles in the *Vita* the reader needs to be familiar with the symbolism of *The Prophecies of Merlin* (analysed in the above book), but this is not essential for the psychological transformative and magical themes of individual growth and maturity that form the core of the narrative.

In essence *The Life of Merlin* is vast entertainment, a jocular ballad as Geoffrey (the assembler and part author) himself might have termed it. It contains a number of subtle jokes and some well-drawn characters who shine through the long passages of knowledge and wisdom that seem so obscure to the modern reader. As the narrative is obviously assembled from various other poems, bardic fragments and classical texts often repeated very close to the original, I have not hesitated to separate these individual units, and give them sub-titles for purposes of general accessibility.

Many of the qualities and roles undertaken by Merlin are clearly linked to Celtic mythology and to a pagan religion or magical system; they are often quite different from those which he was to assume in the popular field of literature in later centuries. It remains to be established whether or not these qualities were originally attached to Merlin, or if Geoffrey of Monmouth added some of them to his main magical spiritual character for the sake of completeness, drawing them from Celtic tradition in general through his familiarity with Welsh or Breton stories and songs or declamations. *Completeness* was beloved of the medieval mind; the geocentric system, the hierarchies of Church and State, the vision of a future and a Resurrection; all were replete with a sense of order, relationship, and manifestation of clear patterns. Set against this we have the chaotic visions of the pagan seers, sprouting protean shapes from a mystical world-view that was gradually dragged into order through the centuries, yet nevertheless derived from some very sophisticated metaphysics which had influenced the learned men of the medieval culture through classical sources.

In the *Vita* these two streams of symbolism and philosophy are merged; sometimes they alternate just as the magical streams of the World are described as alternating by the bard Taliesin in one of our later chapters; sometimes they flow together in a mixture so rich and inseparable that a third source is felt beyond them both, a source in the mysterious Otherworld.

To support the poetic and imaginative elements revealed, I have added a number of poems and other items as Appendices. These extra delights are mainly old Welsh verses that show striking similarities to images in the *Vita*, or extracts from

early tales that are based upon themes clearly known to
Geoffrey and, most important of all, to his audience. Rather
than assemble a mass of notes regarding the dating and origin
of these items, I have merely indicated wherever possible the
major reference works in which this evidence may be found in
great detail. It must be sufficient here to state that the various
verses and tales are not necessarily derived from the *Vita*, and
that the *Vita* is not necessarily derived from them or their lost
'originals'. In an essentially oral story-telling tradition there are
no originals; such creatures only exist in literary terms. Having
said this, I obviously wish to exclude forgeries and reconstruc-
tions, and have added only items which are confirmed as genuine
in one way or another by the authoritative scholarly sources.

The *Vita* is a subtle work, it has many levels; I do not claim
to have plumbed its depths, but merely to have made a series of
soundings along the seaways that it takes. The presence of
complex and harmonic transformative themes (magic and
proto-psychology) is in itself almost baffling: did Geoffrey see
the ancient lore as a coherent pattern? did his noble and
generally illiterate listeners grasp the subtleties of the Celtic
allusions, they being mainly of Norman extraction? did the
bardic sources from whom the legendary magical and prophetic
themes were drawn understand their depth? These are all
questions that were uppermost in my mind when I began this
book. Some of the answers I have given at length in the
following chapters, but others I leave to the reader to make his
or her own judgement.

One thing is certain: I had commenced upon the *Vita* with
the assumption that it was a random jumble of old folkloric
and magical remains mixed with political prophecy . . . a type
of hashed-up second novel to follow Geoffrey's 'best seller' of
The Prophecies. It was only when I began to truly examine the
themes that I realised how intimately they are linked together,
and with what depth and subtlety they are drawn. This depth is
partly lost to the modern reader through the long educational
diversions such as the lists of creatures, springs, birds, and the
like, drawn from sources known to the medieval scholar. We
do not have the attention span of earlier centuries, and we find

these interludes confusing or even irrelevant. I have tried to show that they are very relevant indeed to the deepest spiritual themes of growth, but nevertheless have isolated some of them for the sake of mercy upon the reader.

Geoffrey's poetic narrative is the first literary version of an ancient extended story-telling, known as the Creation of the World and the Adventures of the First and Last Man: a primal everyman personified through Merlin. It is also the last version of this extended organic type of telling, for it froze the theme into literature, having a profound effect upon all literature that was to follow. This conclusion applies also to the greater book of *The History of the British Kings*, which includes *The Prophecies*; they are watersheds in the transition from oral tradition to written literature, even though they are not historically by any means early in terms of setting tales into written chronicle form. It is the style and most of all the content that marks these works, and nowhere is the proto-psychology, magic, and spiritual theme of growth more clearly developed than in the *Vita*.

Merlin finally outgrows even his own prophetic powers; he turns entirely to spiritual contemplation, and a vision of a life attuned to the Divine closes the narrative after lengthy and mainly pagan expositions and adventures. Some scholars have suggested that this closing theme is due to Geoffrey's own final appointment as bishop at about the time of writing, and that he was poetically separating himself from his earlier apocalyptic pagan visions of Merlin in the Book of *The Prophecies*. I feel that the *Vita* is a work of such depth that this would be a trivial reason for Merlin's final devotion to the life of the spirit and his prayers to a more transcendent divinity than the UnderWorld powers and the fervent woodland god. The conclusion of the *Vita* is a spiritual ending totally in keeping with the great philosophies and religions worldwide: unconsciousness seeks to attune only to the divine, the unknown, the creator, the source. Magical powers are merely one way towards this attune-ment or atonement, but it is this very specific way that Merlin takes, and *The Life of Merlin* is a powerful model for the inner life of the developing psyche.

Finally I would like to point out that the *Vita* is a very effective and powerful piece of story-telling; it is the stuff of active dreams, and strikes notes that remind us repeatedly of melodies almost lost, but never quite forgotten. If we read and enter into this *Life of Merlin*, we begin to dream these dreams, to hear these Otherworldly melodies, to see the visions so clearly described by Merlin and Taliesin in the narrative. But more than that, we add to them, recreate them, and perhaps in time fulfill their timeless promises not only within ourselves, but in the outer world that we create through our imagination.

USING THIS BOOK

The *Vita Merlini* seems horribly complicated to the modern reader approaching it for the first time. As it is an initiatory or magical-spiritual text (plus many other types or categories in addition to this central theme of inner growth) it becomes suddenly clear and lucid once its foundations have been understood.

To help both myself and the reader to come to grips with these foundations, I have made a number of separations, and devised a simple method of dealing with the *Vita* that will be helpful to both the new reader and to those who have already studied the text. The recommendations offered are thus:

1   Read the Conclusions (at the end of this book) before reading the text. When you have read the whole book, they will of course be seen in a different light, but are a good anchoring point before setting out upon the ocean.

2   Next read Appendix II, *People*, to gain some grounding in the rather unusual and multifold characterisation of the main figures in the narrative, then proceed to the Introduction and Chapter 1.

3   Read the short summary of each division at the head of each Chapter, in which the plot of the *Vita* is given as simply as possible. The poetic and other quotations under the Chapter headings are not intended as cross-references, but to set the scene or mood for the division of the *Vita* which follows.

Thereafter you may choose whether or not to read the translated text first, or the commentary first. Both are equally important, for the text works in a subtle and dreamlike manner upon levels of our consciousness that are deep and regenerative; a mere summary or commentary cannot do this. But the commentary and the other Appendices will give our intellects some firm anchoring points; like *Barinthus*, the mysterious guiding being who 'knows the sea and stars' (see Appendix II) the points of the *Vita* that we can understand eventually become a ferryman, fused out of many strange and magical elements, carrying us towards the Otherworld where transformation and revelation are found.

There are continuing cross-references to a set of notes which include the short basic bibliography for further reading; I have intentionally kept the notes and references to a minimum. Many of the reference works listed have extensive bibliographies which are valuable for further study.

THE ILLUSTRATIONS

There are two types of illustration: the first are maps or glyphs, while the second are pictoral symbols. Both are set out in the style of traditional magical or initiatory emblems, not to be quaint or falsely antiquarian, but because such methods are proven and hallowed applications of imagery within the psyche. In the East they would be called *mandalas*, and the basic patterns such as the Wheel of Life are known the world over from the most ancient times to the present day.

The illustrations may be used in two ways: firstly to help in grasping the argument or description in the text; secondly as meditative glyphs or images in their own right. This second method should be followed by those readers who wish to take up the practical application of the *Vita* in their own meditations, but the first method is very valuable as a foundation for such further work. There is a list of images in Appendix I which will come alive for the imagination with a little effort. Working through the *Vita* has a remarkable effect upon the imagination; in this sense it is a truly magically potent book, for it works directly upon our image-making consciousness. The illustrations in this volume are part of a set with those in *The Prophetic Vision of Merlin*, the companion book which deals with an earlier prophetic set of verses also assembled by Geoffrey of Monmouth.

There is no reason, of course, why you should not merely read the book through from beginning to end, as it is set out in the usual manner in which the argument or theories are developed as the chapters progress. Because of the harmonic nature of the *Vita* in which many motifs and elements relate to one another in a spiralling or non-linear manner, any analysis of the text involves a great deal of hopping back and forward across the connecting strands of the web. In earlier cultures the human memory was considerably more powerful than our electronically buttressed and buffered ability today; the listeners to such magical narratives would have been able to make many of the connections easily that involve much labor for us. They would also have made many connections that I have undoubtedly missed, which perhaps the reader will find.

Acknowledgements

Translations of the *Vita Merlini* employed in this book are based upon the work of John Jay Parry (University of Illinois, 1925) with a number of amendments based upon my own reading of the Latin text published by Basil Clarke (University of Wales, 1973). Clarke is the most recent and comprehensive study and translation of the *Vita*, and both Parry and Clarke provide extensive references and short scholarly commentaries upon obscure aspects of the text. Other translations, such as verses from *The Prophecies of Merlin* or *The History of the British Kings* are by J.A. Giles (1848-96) unless otherwise stated. The divisions, sub-titles, context and amendments of translated passages are my own; the divisions are merely for use in the present book, and are not offered as restorations or definitive textual elements.

I would like to express my gratitude to A.T. Mann and Tony Willis for discussing astrological and astronomical implications of the text; John and Caitlín Matthews for elucidation of personae in *The Mabinogion*; Felicity Bowers for the original illustrations based upon my own crude sketches. Acknowledgement is also due to the many friends and co-workers who have helped my understanding of the *Vita* through a diverse network of experience and communication, enlivening the more academic or literary sources, and transforming the subject into a matter of humanity rather than mere linguistics.

MERLIN INVOKES BARINTHUS

Who knows well the way of sea and stars?
Who the strong hand upon the helm of passage?
Who guides the keel that ploughs the deep?
First ferryman, last light-bringer,
Blue cloak, white hair;
Wave tops are your pathway,
Starlight your compass.
I who have been within your vessel
Not once but many times from star to star,
Bid you enter.
Oldest of the guiding gods
Wisest of the deep lords,
Eternal sea ruler.
Open is the Western Gate
Where the assembled company of worlds
Awaits the passenger you bring.

R.J. Stewart, 1985

Introduction

He drew the following illustrations under the guidance of Minerva.

Vita Merlini.

INNER TRANSFORMATION AND THE *VITA MERLINI*

Western esoteric traditions retain powerful methods of psychic magical and spiritual transformation. Such insight and wisdom is not the exclusive property of Eastern culture, as has been falsely assumed and taught in many schools of modern psychology and transpersonal development. The wisdom teachings of the West, however, require a fresh assessment of both their vocabulary and their means of employment for the individual or the group in pursuit of inner transformation.

No figure represents this wisdom more strongly than Merlin, the primal seer, prophet, and enlightened wise man of British and Western legends. If we wish to restore a practical system of Western psychic growth, based upon traditional lore, we cannot do better than to work with the symbols relating to Merlin, his Prophecies, and his life.

Both *The Prophecies* and *The Life of Merlin* remain as literary curiosities, from the pen of the twelfth-century historian and mythographer Geoffrey of Monmouth.[1] *The Prophecies* represent a mixture of political and trans-temporal vision while simultaneously providing a map of the areas of consciousness which originate the power of prophecy itself.[2]

The *Vita Merlini* or *Life of Merlin* is a different and more complex book. Written under patronage, and by popular request, it is the original extensive biography of Merlin, which

1

set the scene for the many tales, legends, and imaginative works that followed through the centuries. Both *The Life* and *The Prophecies* are remarkable books, for they encapsulate certain obscure but enduring traditions: the wisdom teachings of the West which provide keys to our innate spiritual heritage. This is expressed clearly in the poetry, art, music, and literature developed from the Merlinic and Arthurian themes, but goes far deeper than the famous master-works themselves, and enables us to pursue spiritual illumination and expansion of consciousness by very specific methods. As these are the methods natural to the Western psyche, they are potent and highly effective in application, giving rapid and often startling results within the consciousness.

In our reassessment of Western techniques and symbols of inner transformation and growth, *The Life of Merlin* plays a vital role. We shall examine the contents of Geoffrey's strange biography, and discover how they relate to many symbols, images, methods and modes of consciousness. Indeed, many of the garbled and ineffective elements of modern esoteric or occult literature are clarified by an understanding of both *The Prophecies* and *The Life*. *The Life of Merlin* is particularly valuable in this context.

The material set out by Geoffrey is not a biography in the modern sense, nor was it ever intended as such. It is a collection of traditional tales, images, poems, and loosely related themes, all woven around the central figure of Merlin. While our medieval text is a unique work of literature, it is not imaginative fiction. The contents of the *Vita Merlini* derive from a number of sources which predate its assembly; it is an anthology.[3] The juxtaposition and interconnection of various elements is extremely subtle, and works on many different levels which we shall examine as we explore the specific contents. Furthermore, the effect of combining these diffuse but harmonically related elements through the hand of one author, Geoffrey, is that of a time-capsule. We have been sent, through the centuries, the basic lore of an oral wisdom tradition, assembled at a time when that tradition was waning but by no means defunct.

The imagery, magical and psychic methods of insight, and the spiritual viewpoint of the *Vita*, are undeniably ancient. Although the wisdom teachings are often obscured by mistranslation (having come from Welsh or Breton into Latin and on to the modern reader in various English translations) and are mixed with derivative or even irrelevant material from medieval convention, they may be reasonably defined as 'Druidic'. By this we should understand that they derive from the original teachings of the primal religions of the West, especially those of the Celts, whose cult practices were formally led by the Druids. This Druidic and Celtic lore is intermixed with classical Greek and Roman material, though much of this is a literary convention on the part of Geoffrey, and not necessarily a cultural or magical line of enduring symbolism.

The lore of Merlin comes from an oral tradition in which the written word was originally unknown and later repudiated, as an enervating influence upon consciousness. By the twelfth century, when both Geoffrey of Monmouth and Gerald of Wales were collecting Celtic prophecies, the ancient poems were still widespread, but in a very confused and decadent state. Gerald tells us that he could not find anyone able to make an adequate translation of a written collection of the predictions circulated by word of mouth among the Welsh bards.[4] Geoffrey, however, was a Welsh or Breton speaker (both languages being similar if not identical in the twelfth century) and there is a continuing dispute over his sources, which he claimed to be a great book in the 'British tongue'.

The oral tradition is essentially practical and intimate, not intellectual or formally educational in the modern sense. Many of the spiritual or wisdom elements are preserved in poetry, songs, tales and customs which endured not only into the medieval period, but survived changes of culture and language, and persisted in a concentrated form well into the twentieth century. Such tradition devolves to us from a heroic 'shamanistic' and mystical culture, in which the profound depths of both collective and individual imagination were given expression through a fluid alphabet of interlinked symbols.

Much of this culture, which we loosely define as Celtic,

persists to the present day, and should not be regarded as a curiosity or escapist fantasy based upon the lost past. The powerful motivations of our ancestors live on within us, and may yet come alive to transform our consciousness. Significantly, this transformation is in the manner of a mutual exchange, for we, by activating the ancient keys to a transformed awareness, also refine the atavistic elements inherent in the primal symbols. They energise us, we purify and carry them forward to a unified future. It was through this experience that Merlin was able to foretell events accurately.[5]

Many of the main symbols found in the *Vita Merlini* are still present in the confused body of literary occultism, most of which derives from the complex flourishing of interest in esoteric matters in the late nineteenth and present twentieth centuries. Some of this modern material is founded upon alchemy, Qabalah, Renaissance theosophy (as opposed to the nineteenth-century movement) and continuing traditions which fused classical and non-classical religion, magic, and metaphysics. Very little of the literary work on Western esoteric methods, however, goes to the fundamental source of Merlin; most 'occult' writers are sadly ignorant of the very existence of both *The Prophecies* and *The Life*. A good example of this enduring symbolism will be discussed Chapter 5, in which the Tarot image of the Hanged Man is clearly seen to be related to a description found in the *Vita*, while this in turn is derived from an ancient sacrificial theme which runs through all mystical insight and many formal religions.

Modern occultism, lamentably ill informed, suggests many sources for the Tarot images, yet a number of the Major Arcana are clearly described by Geoffrey of Monmouth in his setting out of oral wisdom tales or poems from Celtic tradition.[6] The images, therefore, are present in the shared imagination *and* in the 'Druidic' teachings at least as early as the fifth to twelfth centuries, which is the period defined by scholars for the general ambience of Geoffrey's native sources. The cultural patterns, of course, are more ancient, and were known to the Greeks and Romans as being typically Celtic, well before the Christian era.

In the *Vita Merlini* we find many self-contained episodes which have derived from oral use; Geoffrey would have found them as poems, songs, declamations, or tales circulated widely in the Celtic regions of Brittany, Wales, Scotland, and the Western parts of England. They form, ostensibly, a biography of Merlin, and give details of his predictions, his fits of prophetic fervour, his ritualistic and mystical acts and conversations.

The *Vita* is, in one sense, the Celtic equivalent of the Christian New Testament, while Geoffrey's *History of The British Kings* incorporating *The Prophecies* is the equivalent of the Old Testament. This is not an idle comparison, for the *Vita* collects the teaching, sayings, and life pattern of the greatest prophet of the Western world, while *The History* recounts the tribal mythology of the development of his people.

This analogy should not be drawn too tightly, however, for the Celtic consciousness embraced Christianity at a very early date, before the Roman Church developed, and the Christian spiritual enlightenment is part of the unified consciousness accessible to the seeker of the Grail. It is this very unification, in which the pagan magic and the Christian vision are fused together, that is the hallmark of the Celtic and Western enlightenment.[7]

We shall be examining, therefore, a fluid set of images and parables with a teaching element that is not incorporated in the orthodox framework of a specific religion. Nor do the visions, poems, fragments and allegories ever pretend to issue as dogmatic utterances from the mouth of one master, for they are loosely arranged as a narrative told by a chronicler, though often reverting to the first person of Merlin or one of his relatives or associates. It is Merlin, nevertheless, who merges these elements together, through long-standing traditional association in the Western consciousness as the epitome of all who are transformed inwardly by mystical power.

Before embarking upon the practical applications of Merlin's lore within the modern psyche, we must first understand that his use of pagan magic is not in pursuit of self-aggrandisement. He is not an 'adept' in the modern sense of the superman of

Nietzsche or Crowley, or of the elitist type often associated with secretive 'magical orders'. We must dispose of this type of juvenile nonsense utterly if we are to gain true insight and transformation. The tales which surround Merlin, and the greater cycles of the Arthurian legends and the Grail Quest, all give very clear glimpses of the varied signposts upon the spiritual path. As we are concentrating upon one particular and primal enlightenment, that of Merlin, the greater mass of Arthurian lore is deliberately set aside unless it has specific relevance to an aspect of our exploration.

According to both the *Vita* and *The Prophecies*, and the biographical material in *The History*, Merlin's powers are not magical in the trivial sense. They are found to be cyclical, related to the energies of the land, mysterious at times even to the prophet himself, and at the service of his people. We shall deal in detail with these aspects in the following chapters, as they arise in the analysis of the main themes and motifs in the *Vita*. While the imagery and methods are occasionally similar to those of the Amerindian medicine man or woman, or the Siberian shaman or shamanka, it is the mystical insight and prophetic understanding linked to spiritual illumination that hallmark the character of Merlin. He is a spiritual being, transformed from the human state into a higher mode of consciousness, yet still human.

We are all spiritual beings according to the wisdom teachings, but most of us do not make the transition of active consciousness from our present limited state into one of inner freedom. Merlin is not a mere exhibitor of paranormal abilities, and to approach his methods of enlightenment in this manner is to risk madness . . . one of the very clear parables which we shall encounter shortly.

Just as Merlin's magic is very different from the modern misconception of so-called occultism, so is his madness different from our concepts of insanity or mental imbalance. To place Merlin's radical change of consciousness into a modern context, we must consider it in two specific ways, neither of which necessarily refers to an actual illness or maladaptive period. Firstly, Merlin is a symbolic model of transformed consciousness; his movements and his utterances are highly amplified, even exaggerated, archetypified. Secondly he acts through this representation as a guiding image for individual or collective inner analysis; we are not 'mad' to pursue unworldly ends or to change the direction of our flow of awareness, but we are following the path of Merlin. The person who meditates, perceives with a heightened imagination, or seeks actual withdrawal from society (a rare occurrence in the West) is 'mad' by materialist standards. As we shall see shortly, he or she was regarded thus even in medieval times, and a person who was taken up by spiritual withdrawal or heightened consciousness was regarded traditionally as dead . . . which is to say, dead to one world but alive to another.

Like any concentrated transformative agent, be it physical, emotional, or transpersonal and metaphysical, the methods of initiation can be disturbing and difficult. But life is disturbing and difficult, and whereas the trials of human life revolve in a closed circle, the trials of initiation expand in a spiral. This theme is repeatedly demonstrated by Merlin's own life, where he progresses through his grief to madness, and through his madness to a spiritual maturity and a new form of sanity. We should not, therefore, dread that the traditional methods of transforming the awareness will lead us to imbalanced health or maladaptive behaviour, for those same methods give us a clear and firmly orientated path to follow which leads to a balanced and transformed consciousness. Merlin demonstrates each stage of this inner journey through his own adventures.

The madness of Merlin is merely a stage through which he passes, and it is derived from his material condition of grief, suffering, guilt or compassion. His madness, therefore, is an amplification of our perpetual and collective madness in which we never ask the true questions regarding life, and so repeat our follies endlessly. Some of these questions are found uttered and answered in the *Vita*, though the answers are often surprising and multifold. Arousal of inner energies plays an important part in Merlin's cycle of transformation, but equally important is the resolution, polarising, and harmonisation of those same energies.

We should approach the *Vita Merlini* as a pool or fluid source of enlightenment and inspiration; like the Otherworld cauldron or magical fountains of the Celts (a theme encountered directly in both *The Life* and *The Prophecies*), its contents can both kill and cure. If absorbed correctly, they lead to psychic and spiritual growth; if misapplied they are sources of deadly corrosion and inner death. Fortunately the instructions for safety and for balanced use are included, engraved as it were, upon the rim of the cauldron. If we choose to ignore them that is our own folly, and not the fault of the vessel itself.[8]

Into the pool of motifs, fragments of wisdom teaching, and clearly defined units of magical method and vision, are drawn elements from diffuse sources. Some are parallelled in folklore magic and religion worldwide, for they are common properties of human consciousness, but all are stamped with a uniquely Western characteristic. This clear and unfailingly recognisable hallmark is as follows:

> *Spiritual growth is an individual and non-religious*
> *transformation.*

As suggested above, this does not preclude Christianity or debar religion in any way, but it is the central method of inner development within the Western Mysteries. Merlin is the grand master of these Mysteries, the final image and innerworld being in a holistic pattern of harmonic consciousness ranging through our psychic constructs, images, archetypes, ancestors, and highly charged imaginative contacts with innerworld mediators and spiritual teachers.

Before moving into the remarkable imaginative landscape of Merlin's magical Wales (a Wales both historical and symbolic) we must realise that the material that we encounter therein is not an entire or closed system. If the lore of Merlin were a 'complete' spiritual system, it would be a fossil or a fraud. The completion is found within ourselves, and wholeness is an organic process that operates in varied ways according to each of us. The incomplete and paradoxical nature of Geoffrey's books and material on Merlin is not merely a matter of literary confusion, although this clearly plays a part. It is an inherent property of all spiritual or mystical progressions, for *we* are the end result, we remake the teachings and find wholeness thereby; they do not, and cannot, mould us according to some sterile dogmatic pattern.

This remaking of ourselves, which is the remaking of the world, and in religious terminology the return of the Saviour or Second Coming, is central to the wisdom of Merlin. In his *Prophecies* we find the dramatic apocalyptic vision of the end of the solar system; in *The Life* we find a clear description of the creation of the worlds, from the stellar realms and primary Four Elements to the manifestation of humankind and the planet. Both of these visions are quite consistent with medieval orthodoxy, and so are not remarkable for their presence in a collection of legendary history or vaticinal literature. They are, however, unorthodox in their content, tone, and religious attitude. Neither, for example, can be said to be utterly 'Christian', while the vision of the end of time in *The Prophecies* has a totally pagan Celtic and semi-classical symbolism, almost as if the Church did not exist.[9]

The Creation vision from *The Life* is remarkably close to certain esoteric teachings upon the nature of the worlds, and is uttered under the guidance of Minerva, the classical goddess of culture, development of society, music, scientific invention, and the patroness of many significant heroes upon their magical and spiritual quests. As we shall discover later, Minerva is merely the initial magical or goddess image for an important sequence of female innerworld powers, and the use of her name was a convention which defined a deeper and culturally widespread divinity.[10]

Although we remake the worlds, according to Merlin, we may not do this wilfully. There is a paradox inherent in the Western Mysteries, which runs through all mystical experience. The inner ferment and transformation is catalysed by images from the shared imagination; these are known to us as the figures of Merlin, Arthur, The Tower, the Dragons, the Fountain and many more. Some of these images represent actual persons who had a historical life, while others are utterly archetypal; but all are charged with a remarkable potency that awaits release within ourselves.[11]

These catalysing images work upon certain combined elements of imagination and life energy; none of the process is sterile or merely mental. A simple summary of the interaction is difficult, for many variable factors are involved, but the individual requires the containing structure of the tradition; this structure acts as a vessel of restraint upon the conscious-ness. In alchemy, the materials for the Great Work are contained within an alembic or specially sealed vessel, and this has parallels with mystical consciousness.[12] It is the enclosing and applied inheritance of the Western esoteric tradition that provides the matrix or vessel that leads to liberation. A modern analogy is that of the space-craft, employing some very basic physical laws that hold good even in the realms of conscious-ness. Tremendous energies are encapsulated in a vessel, which thrusts against a collection of restraining influences (the walls, the engine-blocks, the launching gantry or pad, and the planet itself). These influences are so arranged that the end result can only be a lifting clear of the surface and a liberation into a new dimension: physical extra-terrestrial space.

This is not a new discovery by any means, and as a basic law of physics it has been employed as a teaching guide in the Mysteries since the days of Pythagoras or Plato, and probably long before. While we use our current technology to illustrate the analogy, the ancients employed the laws of acoustics, geometry, and other physical systems directly within their culture.[13] However the model is arranged, the analogy is clear; *consciousness is liberated through certain harmonic sets of restrictions.*

These are the basic disciplines required in meditation, visualisation, healthy living and self restraint, but this is merely the first expressive level of the controlling structure. The outer expression derives from an inner and imaginative world, which is always represented, worldwide, by collective traditions that reach far into the human and environmental matrix, where the poetic past creates the potential future.[14]

The Western psyche is most actively transformed by the natural matrix of the West; this matrix is precisely what we encounter in the lore of Merlin.

In other words, we must accept, live, and breathe, the traditional symbols, images, patterns, modes of consciousness, and enter into them in meditation, imagination, and creative activity, whenever possible.

This seems, superficially, like an immense charge upon the individual who leads a computer and video-bound life in the metropolis; but the first restrictive path to liberation is always one of self-discipline. If we are able to spend a short amount of time regularly in attuning to the transformative traditions (by reading, music, poetry, visualisations and meditation) they come alive with surprising speed within our consciousness. This rapid response is due to the simple fact that we are merely reawakening slumbering elements of our inherent psychic and spiritual nature, and this is the beginning of a remarkable and liberating sequence of experiences.[15]

The experiences referred to are not restricted to the imagination; as the imagination creates the outer world, so will our relationship to the Mysteries transform our outer lives.

CHAPTER 1
The outer structure and inner nature of the Vita Merlini

The *Vita Merlini* may be initially defined as an exoteric or outer-seeming entertainment, with an esoteric or inner meaning that underpins the more obvious levels of direct story-telling. But the interrelationship between the outer structure and the inner nature is an organic one; we cannot merely remove the outer layer and peer inside. Before dealing with the narrative in detail we can make an introductory separation of the two levels, but we must always bear in mind that this dissection is merely an artificial and convenient starting point, a dip into the pool before we plunge into the deeper waters of the *Vita* itself.

When Merlin asks 'What is the meaning of weather?' in a later chapter, he is answered by a description of the entire cosmos, so when we ask about the meaning of the *Vita* which includes this question, we can hardly expect simplistic answers. The narrative, like many mystical texts and teachings, is full of connectives: symbols and relationships which in turn lead to further relationships. It is indeed the cosmos that causes weather, but as inhabitants of one planet, Earth, we need mundane starting points to help us grasp the greater vision of reality.

THE OUTER STRUCTURE

The structure of the *Vita Merlini* is complex: the narrative poem contains a series of pseudo-historical events, persons, and places, in which magical and mystical motifs are embedded. To

13

grasp the subtle roots of its meaning is not merely a matter of extracting the major motifs and analysing them – many of the most valuable symbols are found as mere asides in narrative context.

We shall be considering the contents from a psychological, magical and mystical viewpoint, so the historical and literary discussions are only touched upon where they have direct relevance to a particular theme.

The *Vita* opens, for example, with a battle between the North Welsh and the Scots; this has been given a historical context which scholars date to the battle of Arderydd, fought near Carlisle in about AD 575. The psychological and magical implications of this battle are more important to us than the historical correlation, for it was in this conflict that Merlin was driven mad. Madness is a recurring theme in Celtic lore, and does not carry the stigma that insanity bears today. The breakdown of regular serial cognition is part of mystical insight, and the historical battle is really a corroborative expression of a widespread motif in which conflict of opposing energies brings on a radical change of consciousness.

This theme is repeated at greater length in *The History*, shortly before *The Prophecies* are uttered by Merlin. The warring powers are represented by two dragons, which in turn stand for the British and the Saxons, but clearly imply energies both from within the earth and from the depths of the human psyche. The historical element is present here also, for the Saxons did invade Britain, but the metaphysical realities are always apparent as a foundation for the physical and historical expressions.[1]

Having reached this far in our perception of the link between outer expression and poetical or mystical powers, we find that the entire pattern of interwoven history and metaphysics runs through Geoffrey's books, and is clearly not a contrivance but a property of the traditional style which he is adapting into his Latin text. Put simply, the poetic powers create history: the prophetic insight is not merely 'confirmed' by accurate 'events', it is unified with those events in a dimension or state that obviates serial time. Imagination is always breaking through into outer expression; eventually we gain the insight that history merely confirms the reality of the inner consciousness, and not vice versa.

This important teaching, therefore, is spread through the *Vita Merlini*, *The Prophecies*, and *The History*; it derives from a world-view typical to the Celts, and central to the Western Mysteries.

Within the broad framework of physical/poetical interaction, we can approach the *Vita Merlini* and extract some of the most effective magical images and techniques that lead to mystical insight. In all cases demonstrated, the magical operation (or psychological transformation) is a means towards mystical or spiritual enlightenment; it is never gratuitous or merely experimental, it is always attuned and defined.

Merlin undergoes some devastating life experiences; he is driven insane, he cannot support himself in the woods in winter, his wife leaves him, many of his companions are killed by misuse of magical powers. These and other themes will be considered in detail, but the implication is that of forces that transform and amplify the regular flow of consciousness. There is no moral suggestion of punishment in these motifs; Merlin is undergoing cycles of change, and the tales that express those cycles must be read as allegories of our inner condition.

To balance these apparently negative experiences, we find that Merlin has powers of far-seeing, prophecy, poetry, star-lore, and that he eventually understands the secret powers of the Earth expressed through fountains, trees, stones, and forests. Once again, we must see not only the physical picture but its psychic and spiritual origination.

Many of the significant elements in the *Vita* were clearly independent images or tales before they were set in context by Geoffrey; some of them are connected to the persona of Merlin in a manner which seems at first contrived.[2]

In certain cases, the magical and mystical lore does not centre upon Merlin but on other characters in the poem, some of them quite minor or anonymous. The thread which weaves these units together is Merlin's prophetic fervour, his fits of madness. He is, therefore, a powerful unifying focus of consciousness.

As mentioned above, the central thesis of the Western Mysteries is that the primal spirit creates outer reality through imagination. In the individual this has its most dramatic expression in the prophetic insight which causes time and events to coalesce. When we find examples of this in profusion through Geoffrey's work, we are not merely encountering literary contrivance, but a poetic expression of a mystical world-view; *inspiration creates reality through imagination.*

This conceptual model must not be readily applied to make Merlin into a god-like figure: there is no implication that prediction forces future events. The predictive or vaticinal powers are not causative or at the command of the individual personality. Merlin is not ordering fate when he predicts The Threefold Death for a youth at the court of King Rhydderch.[3] He is giving verbal expression to a spiritual and imaginative matrix that transcends serial perception of time; the matrix that creates both the 'event' and the 'seeing' of the event.

This insight or farsight embraces both factual and mundane patterns and recondite symbolic relationships, for both derive from the same inner source. History is an expression of poetry, and not vice versa.

In the example of the youth's mysterious fate, the tale of an unfaithful wife and the testing of a seer's ability becomes the framework for a primal magical and spiritual image. Merlin's prediction, therefore, is merely a peg on which to hang a traditional wisdom tale or initiatory theme; but this may in turn devolve from an older story cycle now lost, in which Merlin plays a more specific role. In *The Prophecies*, however, we find a strong factual element, where precise events and historical persons are suggested. Such prophecies also occur as part of the *Vita*.

When pseudo-historical predictions or retrospective memories appear in the *Vita* they are employed by Geoffrey as corroboration and 'evidence' for the validity of his biography. The use of such passages also breaks up the poetic narrative, and provides support for themes that are utterly in the realm of myth or magic, giving a material or apparently factual expression to dream-like themes such as the sojourn of Arthur in the Fortunate Isle.[4] While we should not regard these prophetic passages as mere 'padding', they are of less value to us than the traditional material into which they have been inserted.

In *The Prophecies* a chaotic and expansive tapestry of mystical apocalyptic and pseudo-historical verses dwells neatly packaged within the longer text of *The History of the British Kings*, acting as a type of support for the latter, but also including many esoteric, visionary, and astrological symbols which play no part in *The History* at all. In the *Vita* the transpersonal magical adventures and transformations of Merlin offer us an allegory in which the symbols of *The Prophecies* are applied to human life. The potent and often confusing lore of prophetic power is made more accessible through its action in Merlin's own experiences.

The prophetic verses found in the *Vita* are only a minor aspect of the spectrum of *The Prophecies*, and the various verses that are assembled by Geoffrey from oral tradition and his own learning could stand quite well without the prophetic interludes. The *action* of prophecy, however, is important to the narrative, more important in the growth of Merlin towards a mature spiritual consciousness than the contents of any pseudo-history that he utters.

Many of the historical utterances are connected to matters which would have been of great interest to Geoffrey's listeners but are not enduring in terms of psychological or magical symbolism; they are contemporary items of value to the true historian or literary researcher. Such passages do contain images drawn from or supportive of traditional themes, so we cannot be too dismissive of any specific part of the *Vita*; it is a complex organic work in which levels of relationship are continually interacting.

The outer structure of the *Vita Merlini* is therefore a collection of both traditional and literary fragments carefully aligned into an organic text in which we can sometimes detect the hand of Geoffrey of Monmouth writing directly for his audience and repeating items which he knows are popular and politically significant. The bulk of the poem, however, is a polished written form of an elongated story-telling or ballad-singing entertainment; the type of event which held the fabric of society together through shared images, lessons, and familiar ethical traditional instruction. This aspect of the *Vita* cannot be stressed too strongly; it should never be forgotten or under-estimated by the modern scholar or general reader who lives very far removed from a culture in which oral communication and tradition was paramount, with literacy the property of a learned special class to which Geoffrey of course belonged.

We should also remember that the spiritual aspects of the narrative have a firmly stated and overt level of instruction; the *Vita* is not merely a funny collection of old tales that reveal inner values through modern analysis. The poem would have been exemplary or deliberately instructional for Geoffrey's audience, and this is part of its value and appeal to the medieval listener. Many of the aspects of this overt spiritual symbolism are dealt with in our following chapters, but the most significant is that Merlin eventually becomes cured of prophetic madness and retires to a life of spiritual devotion in praise of the Creator.

If this were all that happened in the *Vita* it would, perhaps, not be worth a fresh assessment; but within the overtly spiritual tone there is a great wealth of ancient lore, magical symbolism and quite practical methods of psychic transformation which were probably inherent in the sources from which Geoffrey drew.

We cannot guess at his reasons for setting this material out, they are perhaps reasons of a poetical and intuitive nature, not really subject to mere intellectual analysis. Similar magical themes are found within folk ballads preserved in oral tradition well into the twentieth century, and they remained alive because of the primal power and dream value that they hold.

The *Vita*, however, contains not only visions from the collective dream-pool, but themes, motifs, and Celtic language terms which clearly imply the presence of a coherent wisdom system; a system which is likely to have originated in part with the Druids.[5] What is so remarkable is that the coherence shines through Geoffrey's Latin narrative assembly, though it is most unlikely that he would have written the work with such a coherence fully in mind. The outer structure and characterisation of the *Vita* is full of harmonic and polarised relationships and scenes; they are there in the text right on the surface, and need very little exposition to be apparent. These are underpinned by the implied sub-textual matter, the inner symbolism which is found in the Celtic language names, the strange ambiguities of behaviour, and the key values of apparently minor figures around whom the action obviously revolves at certain points of development.

THE INNER NATURE

The *Vita Merlini* is a comprehensive mystical psychology. Unlike its companion book *The Prophecies*, it does not reveal vast chaotic cosmic visions or pose intense magical paradoxes; it develops in an orderly, almost inevitable manner and leaves very little to chance. This does not imply that the *Vita* is in any way dull, for it vibrates with the poetry and imagery of the relationship between the spiritual and Otherworlds and the personal psyche; it is a mystical psychology and not a materialist one. But psychology it is, for the *Vita* employs the adventures of Merlin to demonstrate a deep and effective understanding of the human psyche.

Even if we take the matter no further than the basic psychic and personal problems expressed and characterised, the *Vita* has many remarkable insights to offer. It is one of the earliest books on the growth and harmonisation of the elemental psyche, employing a cycle of breakdown and restructuring closely related to individual, sexual, and social issues which are, and always will be, significant to human culture.

We find the figure of Merlin symbolising the wild and unpredicatable aspects of human nature, yet this very unpredictability becomes the way towards accurate prediction. Unlike *The Prophecies*, the predictive material takes a second place, it is used only to support the development of the narrative, and to illustrate several motifs of human psychic frailty. The main theme of the *Vita* is a spiralling journey towards inner maturity, in which both inner and outer situations and places are revisited at different levels of the spiral. This maturity is eventually gained at a level which is not common, and which might seem unnecessary to the modern individual; Merlin passes through grief and compassion to liberation from sexual stereotypes to accurate prevision and finally to an ordered conceptual model of the cosmos in which mystical vision, myth, and physical expression are fused together harmoniously. Having reached this state, his original imbalance is cured, and he relinquishes all of his supernormal powers.

This last act of Merlin's is significant; the supernormal aspects of consciousness are merely side-effects and not ends in themselves. The original source of the Merlin material is Western, primarily Celtic, yet we can find striking parallels between this exposition of individual consciousness and the central themes of Buddhism. There is no implication whatsoever that the Merlin legends are drawn from a Buddhist source; the similarities are due to shared qualities of consciousness expressed in myth and religion worldwide. Like the Buddha, Merlin is a prince with every material benefit; he is driven into the woods through grief and compassion at a dreadful battle; he seeks answers to the most basic eternal questions. Like Jesus, he is carried off and tempted by a most worldly and seductive power which he refuses to accept: he rejects the superficial aspects of sexuality or sensuality.[6] But Merlin achieves a harmonious polarised relationship with feminine principles, a major theme of the *Vita*. Like Mohammed, he has visions that trascend time and space. We could draw such comparisons at length and quite fruitlessly, for they prove nothing other than the obvious fact that such traditions of transpersonal and spiritual growth or education are known in every religion, belief, or psychological system.

Due to the ancient Celtic themes which provide a rich foundation for the *Vita*, further comparisons could be made with primal or primitive magical practices, well represented in other early texts, folklore, and the copious studies of anthropology. Authors have been tempted, particularly in recent years, to link Celtic magical lore and the figure of Merlin to 'shamanism', as a result of the similarities mentioned above. This type of labelling, however, begs the question of the sophisticated nature of the *Vita*, and tends to lead us along false paths. If the lore of Merlin is closely connected to shamanism as researched in recent years, then so are all religions, all cults, all magical practices. The comparison, in this sense, must be invalid due to its immense general nature. Furthermore, if we are precise in our use of the term, shamanism does not, and never has, encompassed the areas dealt with in depth in the *Vita*, despite a number of correspondences which are analysed in our main text.[7]

The qualities of the *Vita* are a fusion of two major elements: pagan Celtic and pagan classical. This is perhaps surprising in a period of intense religious orthodoxy (the twelfth century) and very little Christian symbolism or dogma is found in the text of either the *Vita* or *The Prophecies*. Both lines of descent, Celtic and classical (mainly Greek), have certain themes in common, and both reach back through an immensely long period of cultural development, fruition, and decay. There are many influences at work in the *Vita*, but all are firmly pointed in one direction, and under one well-defined systematic mystical psychology. They aim towards the maturity of Merlin, in every sense of the word.

The result is a handbook, an exemplar, which still holds many insights and practical applications for the modern man or woman seeking psychic transformation.

Far from being an obscure literary curiosity, the *Vita Merlini* is one of the great psychological and spiritual expositions, cutting across cultural and geographical barriers. It speaks to us with the same timeless language and employs the same potent methods as other wisdom-texts which are better publicised.

The conclusion of the *Vita* is a remarkable synthesis of mystical symbolism and practice, transcending mere religious orthodoxy. Merlin, the epitome of the pagan seer, grows beyond the supernormal powers of his seership, and achieves an integrated understanding of the universe. He then declares that he will devote his life to spiritual meditations, and that the mantle of prophecy has passed from him. In modern usage, there is more than enough practical mystical magical and psychological knowledge to meet the student who approaches the *Vita* as a handbook of inner development. This material is derived from a fusion of pagan and Christian beliefs, and transcends sectarian limitations in the same manner that the great teachings of Christ or Buddha resound worldwide. Nor is this a grandiose or over-enthusiastic claim; Merlin's wisdom covers the same area of teaching as those known perennially to be the paths to truth.[8]

The value to the modern student of inner disciplines or the seeker after enlightenment is that the methods of Merlin are couched in an entirely Western vocabulary and imagery. They are part of our own natural collective consciousness, and hold the means whereby that consciousness may be transformed either individually or on a larger scale.

To draw out these valuable elements from the narrative of the *Vita*, we must work through the text, which is divided into a related sequence of individual sub-poems, and pause to examine some of the more important symbols and their interconnection within a simple but powerful map of Merlin's travels through his mythical land. Merlin and the land are quite direct analogues of humankind and consciousness, but with the added metaphysical level of analogy between earth and stars.

CHAPTER 2
I *Merlin and madness*
II *The Battle Lament*

Therefore shall the mountains be levelled as the valleys, and
the rivers of the valleys shall run with blood.

The Prophecies of Merlin.

Merlin is a king, ruling well and seeing into the future, giving
laws to the people of South Wales. He takes part in a war
between the Welsh and the Scots; many men are slain,
including three brothers of King Peredur, Merlin's North Welsh
ally.

Filled with grief, Merlin laments the death of the youths, and
eventually becomes disorientated. He flees to the woods, living
as a wild man, forgetting all human society.

MERLIN AND MADNESS

I am preparing to sing the madness of the prophetic bard,
and a humorous poem on Merlin; pray correct the song,
Robert, glory of bishops, by restraining my pen. For we
know that Philosophy has poured over you its divine nectar,
and has made you famous in all things, that you might serve
as an example, a leader and a teacher in the world. Therefore
may you favor my attempt, and see fit to look upon the poet
with better auspices than did that other whom you have just
succeeded, promoted to an honor that you deserve. For
indeed your habits, and your approved life, and your birth,
and your usefulness to the position, and the clergy and the
people all were seeking it for you, and from this circumstance
happy Lincoln is just now exalted to the stars. On this
account I might wish you to be embraced in a fitting song,

23

but I am not equal to the task, even though Orpheus, and
Camerinus, and Macer, and Marius, and mighty-voiced
Rabirius were all to sing with my mouth and all the Muses
were to accompany me. But now, Sisters, accustomed to sing
with me, let us sing the work proposed, and strike the
cithara.[1]

Well then, after many years had passed under many kings,
Merlin the Briton was held famous in the world. He was a
king and a prophet; to the proud people of the South Welsh
he gave laws, and to the chieftains he prophesied the future.
Meanwhile it happened that strife arose between several of
the chiefs of the kingdom, and throughout the cities they
wasted the innocent people with fierce war. Peredur, king of
the North Welsh, made war on Gwenddoleu, who ruled the
realm of Scotland; and already the day fixed for the battle
was at hand, and the leaders were ready in the field, and the
troops were fighting, falling on both sides in a miserable
slaughter. Merlin had come to the war with Peredur and so
had Rhydderch, king of the Cumbrians, both savage men.
They slew the opposing enemy with their hateful swords, and
three brothers of the prince who had followed him through
his wars, always fighting, cut down and broke the battle
lines. Thence they rushed fiercely through the crowded ranks
with such an attack that they soon fell killed.

THE BATTLE LAMENT

At this sight, Merlin, you grieved and poured out sad
complaints throughout the army, and cried out in these
words, 'Could injurious fate be so harmful as to take from
me so many and such great companions, whom recently so
many kings and so many remote kingdoms feared? O
dubious lot of mankind! O death ever near, which has them
always in its power, and strikes with its hidden goad and
drives out the wretched life from the body! O glorious
youths, who now will stand by my side in arms, and with me
will repel the chieftains coming to harm me, and the hosts

rushing upon me? Bold young men your audacity has taken from you your pleasant years and pleasant youth! You who so recently were rushing in arms through the troops, cutting down on every side those who resisted you, now are beating the ground and are red with red blood!' So among the hosts he lamented with flowing tears and mourned for the men, and the savage battle was unceasing. The lines rushed together, enemies were slain by enemies, blood flowed everywhere, and people died on both sides. But at length the Britons assembled their troops from all quarters and all together rushing in arms they fell upon the Scots and wounded them and cut them down, nor did they rest until the hostile battalions turned their backs and fled through unfrequented ways.

Merlin called his companions out from the battle and bade them bury the brothers in a richly colored chapel; and he bewailed the men and did not cease to pour out laments, and he strewed dust on his hair and rent his garments, and prostrate on the ground rolled now hither and now thither. Peredur strove to console him and so did the nobles and the princes, but he would not be comforted nor put up with their beseeching words. He had now lamented for three whole days and had refused food, so great was the grief that consumed him. Then when he had filled the air with so many and so great complaints, new fury seized him and he departed secretly, and fled to the woods not wishing to be seen as he fled. He entered the wood and rejoiced to lie hidden under the ash trees; he marvelled at the wild beasts feeding on the grass of the glades; now he chased after them and again he flew past them; he lived on the roots of grasses and on the grass, on the fruit of the trees and on the mulberries of the thicket. He became a silvan man just as though devoted to the woods. For a whole summer after this, hidden like a wild animal, he remained buried in the woods, found by no one and forgetful of himself and of his kindred.

MERLIN AND MADNESS

> I am preparing to sing of the madness of the prophetic
> bard, and humorous poem on Merlin.
> *Fatidici vatis rabiem musamque jocasam Merlini cantare
> paro (Vita Merlini, opening line).*

There are two introductory elements before we come to the
major theme of Merlin's prophetic madness: the traditional
element, found in the opening line, punctuated by a personal
dedication to Bishop Robert and a classically styled invocation
of the Muses. Geoffrey returns to the traditional form after this
essential dedication has been made. This pattern (see translation) suggests the oral traditional source from which much of
the *Vita* seems to have been derived.

The cross-fertilisation between the collection of lore from
Celtic traditions and Geoffrey's own wide reading and
imagination is complex, but certain sections stand out as being
drawn from native sources. We might picture Geoffrey not only
relying upon chronicles and classical sources (some now lost to
us) but listening to and noting down poetry and song from
travelling bards and entertainers, who, as both he and Gerald
of Wales tell us, retained and transmitted jocular tales, songs,
and prophecies. In this sense, Geoffrey is one of the first British
'folklore collectors', assembling material that has not been
bettered or even fathomed fully by later and ostensibly more
scientific experts. But his collection contains more than a
jumble of mere curiosities from confused sources.

Merlin is cited as a king and a prophet in his own right,
giving us a quite different tradition from that linking Merlin and
Arthur which is stated in *The History*; once again, we are likely to
be encountering a native tradition or combination of traditions.

> Well then, after many years had passed under many kings,
> Merlin the Briton was held famous in the world. He was a
> king and a prophet . . .

These words are strikingly close to the stock in trade phrases
found in folk-tales the world over, and are a type of formal or

required opening, in the same manner as the modern fairy tale retains the ancient formula of 'Once upon a time, in a land far away, there was a . . .'

The scene is being set for the sudden and dramatic madness, and also for certain motifs or events which occur later in the poem due to the interaction between Merlin's royal status and his fits of insanity.

The madness is a re-statement or alternative expression of the same prophetic fervour shown in *The History* by the incident with the Two Dragons, which occurred with Merlin as a youth, born of a noble maiden and a daemon. Although it seems at first as if Geoffrey is welding two traditions together, something often commented upon by scholars, this is only superficially the case. What arises, in fact, is a double expression of a single theme: consciousness is transformed through interplay of forces, polarity, and on occasions by experience of dire conflict. Both the Dragons and the Battle of the *Vita* represent primal foundations to the prophetic fervour or madness. As a result of apparently irreconcilable conflict, Merlin becomes detached from regular consciousness and plunges into realms of mysterious perception and activity.

The subject of *polarity* is central to mystical, magical, psychological, metaphysical and physical statements or systems relating to the universe, to consciousness, to reality. It is direct experience of the interplay between two polarised powers (dragons, sides of battle, good and evil, sensuality and restraint) that gives rise to a third or originating mode or power. In physics this is shown materially by the result obtained from the combination of factors in an experiment; in meditation or metaphysics it is shown by the attainment of a previously unexperienced level or quality of awareness.

So the traditions relating to Merlin state an essential truth, that his prophetic madness derives from personal experience of the interplay of opposing powers.

There is, however, a progressive element in the *Vita*, not found in the presentation of Merlin in *The History* and *The Prophecies*. During the course of the *Vita*, Merlin develops spiritually from a person driven into the wilds through incomprehension and grief to a prophet choosing an ordered seclusion rather than a royal life of power and honour.

The progression is shown not only by the general development of Geoffrey's loose narrative, but by a number of quite individual internal poems or songs which are likely to be drawn from existing tales, ballads or declaimed poems about Merlin, or about the general growth of inner perception as symbolised by Merlin.

This progressive, even educational, direction is not likely to be merely the result of Geoffrey's own creative imagination; he is reworking a tradition in which wisdom or spiritual growth is exemplified by the life history of one specific individual. Furthermore, that tradition is of Merlin, and was current in various poems or songs at the time of Geoffrey's writing. We may find many worldwide parallels to this oral, educational, spiritual matrix, and must be careful to recognise that it is a very specific type of entity in magical or psychological terms.

Ancient tales may be divided into various groups, from cosmic or primal myths through to semi-historic heroic cycles of activity which are attuned to, but not necessarily identical to, the primal mythology. Merlin's cycle of inner development forms yet another group, that of the initiation or expansion of consciousness exemplified by a seer, magician, bard, shaman, or medicine man. Merlin (or other characters worldwide who fill similar roles) is the most energetic, concentrated and stylised example of a system of inner transformation which is not only accessible to us all, but is inherent in the very nature of our consciousness.

THE BATTLE LAMENT

The reaction that Merlin displays to the conflict is twofold: personal, and compassionate. But in both cases, he represents clearly the human reaction to disasters and war; firstly he asks 'Why me?' and secondly he mourns the fallen heroes who died in battle. In the *Vita* this is clearly defined by a poem, in the form of a lament, typical of Celtic heroic tradition.

This is clearly not the Merlin of great wisdom and far-seeing; it is a very normal man plagued by the griefs and sorrows which plague us all. The battle, or war, is the most obvious expression of inner conflict between opposing powers,manifesting on a tribal or international scale. We should always try to be aware that such conflicts in the outer world are expressions of smaller but no less powerful interactions within ourselves, and of vast interactions in the stellar universe, a subject touched upon by Merlin and Taliesin in their teaching upon the Creation[2] and by Merlin in *The Prophecies* when he described the end of the solar system in graphic and unmistakable terms.

But to draw such inclusive connections is not sufficient; it does not solve the personal reaction to the horrors of evil or conflict in the world. The process of change and higher consciousness is therefore gradual, shown by Merlin's own gradual and sometimes retrograde motion towards a mature enlightenment.

In the *Vita* the death of three brothers of Peredur, Prince of the North Welsh, is the focus for Merlin's grief. Although there is some historical basis for the conflict, we also have a fragment of another tale, which is woven loosely through Geoffrey's *Vita* and *The History*, that of the slain hero or heroes, who will rise again.

The three brothers are buried in a chapel ordered by Merlin in his grief, and this tiny motif is reminiscent of the Grail theme in which a knight, king, or hero lies awaiting rebirth in a magical chapel. Similar folk-tales are told of the great prehistoric mounds in which ancient kings or giants are said to sleep. Later in the *Vita* we find the classic reference to Arthur being carried to the mysterious Island of Apples, or Fortunate Isle, for his long wait and cure.

Merlin's madness is catalysed by his protracted grief; he moves from a state of weeping and mourning lucidity (in which he orders the building of the Chapel and recites the lament poem) into a 'new frenzy' (*novas furias*). In a number of related tales, this madness is rationalised as punishment for the misdeeds of the central character, but this aspect is not present in the *Vita*. There is a tendency for non-Christian wisdom tales and songs to be rationalised into a sin-and-punishment ethic by later chroniclers and commentators who have lost touch with the roots of the material, or alternatively seek to deliberately Christianise it. In both Merlin and the related *Lailoken* and *Suibhne* tales we find a mixture of rationalisation and direct recounting of ancient traditions;[3] for our present purposes it is the madness itself, and the central character's progression through madness to a new and higher order of balance that is important, not any crude notion of punishment.

WILD MAN OF THE WOODS

Finally, he flees to the woods, where he lives as a silvan man, or Wild Man of the Woods. This aspect of the tale works upon several levels, and is a common theme in both mythology and magical practices. We can divide the theme into three different levels, which merge almost imperceptibly with one another.

1 *Psychological or personal* The flight back to nature and from humanity is a well-known and continuing phenomenon which develops from the individual stressed beyond endur-ance in warfare. There are a number of veterans of the Vietnam war in the USA who live to this day in the wilds, as silvan men, exactly as described by Geoffrey when telling of Merlin. The shock and horror of their involvement as young men in a horrible dehumanising war has rendered them unable to be at rest in human society; they return to the heart of nature not in any idealised or pseudo-mystical way, but out of a deep driving necessity to live alone in the woods.

This is not merely a matter of 'forgetting', but a deep polarisation of the soul towards primal life, in an attempt to find the balance destroyed by the evil of war. Such individuals have existed in every land after every war; at one time a number of 'shell-shocked' itinerants from the 1914-18 Great War could be found in the British countryside, sleeping in the woods, living off the land or from begging. These were not tramps or idle drifters, but men forced to remain outdoors and close to the natural sources of life as a result of the bombardment of the trenches; some of them were entitled to officer's pensions.

Many more examples could be cited, but the personal and direct level of Merlin's madness should not be lost in the deeper implications of myth or magic. On a lesser scale, we have all experienced at some time or other a shock or unacceptable event which unbalances our usual pattern of thought and emotion; in this sense Merlin's madness is the ultimate end of the scale of the psyche deranged by trauma.

2 *Transpersonal or magical* The individual may also be driven into the woods as a result of new surges of consciousness, higher levels of awareness breaking through into the regular pattern of life. Traditionally, the seer, magician or inspired man or woman may seek enlightenment and undergo certain dramatic transformations in the wild, sometimes in caves, sometimes on high mountain-tops, and at other times in the greenwood. Merlin, incidentally, undertakes all three locations during his career.

The magician seeks the natural environment, as does the saint or holy man, in order to be free of human contact, to concentrate upon the inner powers of enlightenment. Furthermore, there is an enduring tradition of contact with natural energies, or non-human beings, which may be gained in the most elemental surroundings: beneath the earth, by the sea shore, in the wild woods, on mountain-tops.

The Celtic seers who sought the spirits of Nature or of the Otherworld by retiring from human society are the direct forerunners of the mysterious hermits who give spiritual guidance during the Quest for the Holy Grail. In primal cultures today men and woman still seek magical growth through a direct relationship with nature.

3 *Mythical* In this last and most encompassing sense of the theme, we find Merlin attuned to a widespread pagan god-image. This statement must be taken cautiously, for the three levels described are interwoven, and act as harmonics of one another.

In his actions as Wild Man of the Woods, and as Lord of

the Animals[4] as we shall see shortly, Merlin represents a shadowy but powerful god-form, best known in popular literature by the name of Cernunos (a Roman-Celtic term from inscription), the Horned One.[5] Regrettably, this type of symbolism, drawn from ancient myth and intuition, has been confused and even trivialised by its use in modern revival paganism. Because we find Merlin riding a stag, accompanied by a wolf, and living as a Wild Man, does not automatically mean that we are encountering a firm statement of 'witchcraft'.

Similar motifs are found in the *Mabinogion*, Arthurian legends, and in other Celtic tales, all deriving from a culture in which the modern concept of witchcraft (and even the orthodox religious concept of it) had not been developed.

Such figures are not merely the inheritance of a pagan 'nature religion' as is often stated; they are integral parts of a sophisticated metaphysics and philosophy which was, to a certain extent, held in common by the ancient European cultures. Our modern tendency is to take these elements out of their cultural and religious or metaphysical context.

A second aspect of Merlin as the mythical Wild Man is of course the true spiritual analogy that is drawn. He actually grows through all three stages of the sequence: personal, magical, mythical/spiritual. In Geoffrey's resolution of the tale, drawn from Celtic bardic sources in many places, the resolution is *spiritual*; this same spiritual quality is shown in the rationalisations of the *Lailoken* and *Suibhne* tales, where a saint forgives the mad seer or king towards the close of his fore-doomed life. In the *Vita*, however, there is a curious and positive absence of Christian apologetics or rationalisations and we are reminded of a similar absence in Geoffrey's *Prophecies*.

Either Geoffrey has willfully written out all Christian developments and stylishly maintained the pagan/classical symbolism as an element of contrived antiquity, or else he is preserving earlier oral forms in which the orthodox rationalisations simply are not present.

Merlin's spiritual conclusion or devotion is shared with his

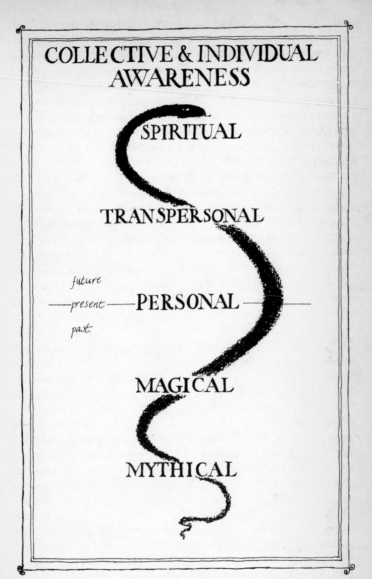

Figure 1 *Collective and individual awareness*

sister,[6] a theme which we shall return to in its proper place, which is at the close of the narrative. It represents the harmonious unity of the masculine and feminine principles, but also shows that both men and women equally may be inspired by spiritual vision.

The three levels of the Wild Man motif also work as three cultural stages through serial or pseudo-historic time. The psychological or personal level corresponds to the present; the transpersonal or magical level corresponds to the collective bardic cultures of early Europe; the mythical/spiritual image corresponds to the primal or orginative past where life-power is known solely as archetypical form.

We might also show this same analogy moving in the polar opposite direction, towards the apparent future (see figure 1) in which the personal present leads into the transpersonal transformative future, which leads in turn to the distant arch-future encompassed by one spiritual entity.

CHAPTER 3
The Winter Lament

The sign-bearing Wolf shall lead.

The Prophecies of Merlin.

After a season living as a wild man close to nature, Merlin
encounters winter. He laments the lack of fruit, nuts, and grass,
and refers specifically to apple trees in a poem which reflects
other Welsh traditional verses that relate incidents from
Merlin's life.

He has a wolf as a companion, but the wolf is dying. A
passerby overhears Merlin's lament, and passes the news on to
a messenger sent by Ganieda (Merlin's sister) to seek for the
mad seer. Merlin is found at the top of a mountain, beside a
fountain or spring.

THE WINTER LAMENT

But when the winter came and took away all the grass and
the fruit of the trees and he had nothing to live on, he poured
out the following lament in a wretched voice.

'Christ, God of heaven, what shall I do? In what part of
the world can I stay, since I see nothing here I can live on,
neither grass on the ground nor acorns on the trees? Here
once there stood nineteen apple trees bearing apples every
year; now they are not standing[1] Who has taken them away
from me? Whither have they gone all of a sudden? Now I see
them – now I do not! Thus the fates fight against me and for
me, since they both permit and forbid me to see. Now I lack
the apples and everything else. The trees stand without
leaves, without fruit; I am afflicted by both circumstances

35

since I cannot cover myself with the leaves or eat the fruit. Winter and the south wind with its falling rain have taken them all away. If by chance I find some roots deep in the ground the hungry swine and the voracious boars rush up and snatch them from me as I dig them up from the turf. You, O wolf, dear companion, accustomed to roam with me through the secluded paths of the woods and meadows, now can scarcely get across the fields; hard hunger has weakened both you and me. You lived in these woods before I did and age has whitened your hairs first. You have nothing to put into your mouth and do not know how to get anything, at which I marvel, since the wood abounds in so many goats and other wild beasts that you might catch. Perhaps that detestable old age of yours has taken away your strength and prevented your following the chase. Now, as the only thing left you, you fill the air with howlings, and stretched out on the ground you extend your wasted limbs.'

These words he was uttering among the shrubs and dense hazel thickets when the sound reached a passer-by who turned his steps to the place whence the sounds were rising in the air, and found the place and found the speaker. As soon as Merlin saw him he departed, and the traveller followed him, but was unable to overtake the man as he fled. Thereupon he resumed his journey and went about his business, moved by the lot of the fugitive. Now this traveller was met by a man from the court of Rhydderch, King of the Cumbrians, who was married to Ganieda and was happy in his beautiful wife. She was sister to Merlin and, grieving over the fate of her brother, she had sent her retainers to the woods and the distant fields to bring him back. One of these retainers came toward the traveller and the latter at once went up to him and they fell into conversation; the one who had been sent to find Merlin asked if the other had seen him in the woods or the glades. The latter admitted that he had seen such a man among the bushy glades of the Calidonian forest, but, when he wished to speak to him and sit down with him, the other had fled away swiftly among the oaks. These things he told, and the messenger departed and entered the forest; he searched the deepest valleys and passed over the high mountains; he sought everywhere for his man, going through the obscure places.

On the very summit of a certain mountain there was a fountain, surrounded on every side by hazel bushes and thick with shrubs. There Merlin had seated himself, and thence through all the woods he watched the wild animals running and playing. Thither the messenger climbed, and with silent step went on up the heights seeking the man. At last he saw the fountain and Merlin sitting on the grass behind it, and making his complaint.

THE WINTER LAMENT

We now come to the second sub-poem, another lament, but of a different and more inward-looking nature. This represents the typical questions that are asked by the individual who looks within, who travels or seeks to travel upon the path towards transformed consciousness, or spiritual enlightenment.

Merlin has spent a summer of madness in the woods, 'forgetful of himself and of his kindred'. This first flush of fury is a type of escape, a brief respite from the tormenting questions that must arise within anyone seeking to grasp or understand the problems of human life. With the arrival of Winter, Merlin asks the questions again, in a new form, but basically related to those asked in the Battle Lament. He complains against the arrival of the season in its due course, he asks 'Why does Winter exist?' His questing consciousness is still childlike, even childish. He represents the individual at the very beginning of the Quest, who cannot find any view that gives insight into the problems of the negative polarities, or the natural power-of-taking.

Just as his first fury and wildness is balanced at the close of the *Vita* by his spiritual retreat accompanied by his sister who will take his place as prophetess, so is this questioning lament answered later by a learned disquisition on the world, the elements, the seasons, and the strange orders of life from the stellar beings through to the inhabitants of the UnderWorld. But before Merlin can receive this complex wisdom teaching, he has to undergo a series of hardships. Winter is the first of these.

In the enduring esoteric traditions, spiritual insight is symbolised by the Circle or Wheel of Life, which corresponds to the Four Seasons of the year. These seasons are harmonically related to the four elements, and the four phases of a human life cycle (see Figure 2). It is Winter which is the most enlightening of seasons, and earth the most spiritual of elements in terms of growth and initiations.

The student of such traditions, be they religious, mystical or magical is usually drawn to the light of Summer, but the experienced or initiated bard, seer, prophet or enlightened individual knows that it is Winter that gives Summer meaning, just as the cold depths of space give a matrix to the radiant stars.

In our human situation, Earth is the most important element, and this is clearly stressed in the *Vita* by Merlin's own progress from incoherent madness to spiritual clarity through his interaction with the seasons and the forces of nature.

MERLIN'S WOLF

During the Winter Lament, we suddenly find that Merlin has an animal companion, an aged wolf. 'You lived in these woods before I did and age has whitened your hairs first.'

This is a hallowed theme, taken from a tradition which is, curiously, no more than stated by Geoffrey. It is possible that the motif was so well known to his listeners, and certainly those who listened to the travelling story-tellers and bards, that it needed no further elaboration. In another source, an old Welsh poem, Merlin addresses a pig; both wolf and pig are native British animals, and represent a magical theme, that of the totem beast.[2]

The wolf was in the woods before Merlin; he therefore represents those wild powers which Merlin found within the

WHEEL OF LIFE

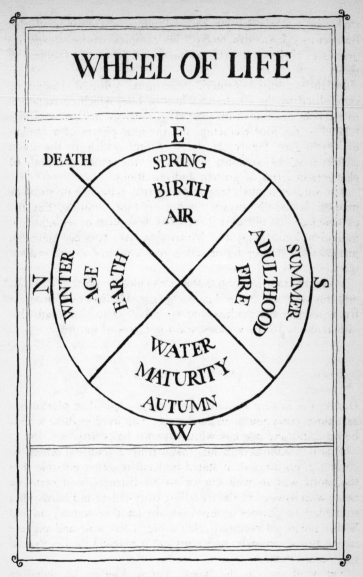

Figure 2 *The Wheel of Life*

woodlands, and in modern psychological terms is an animal symbol for the wild beast within each and every elemental psyche. But spiritual or magical use of animal symbolism is not confined to mere emblems of psychic qualities or behaviour, and the magical beast is employed as an actual entity in many primal magical practices. We find this concept of the beast in the emblems of the Christian saints also, so it is by no means confined to pagan symbolism.

During the development of our analysis of the *Vita*, a number of parallels are found with the symbols on the traditional Tarot cards, a set of pictoral images of unknown origin. The earliest known packs are later than Geoffrey's period by at least two centuries, yet a number of images occur within the *Vita* which are repeated in the Tarot cards. Merlin and his companion wolf are similar to the Fool and his companion dog. Each shows humankind upon the quest, accompanied by a canine animal.

The standard interpretation of this symbolism is that the wolf represents the wild powers of nature or of the psyche being tamed in service of higher ends, just as the dog (in the Tarot symbol) was once wild but has evolved into a tame and faithful guide. This seems to be less than adequate, and the implications of the totem beast and the magical beast are far greater than a mere symbol of presumed evolution or development.

The dog is an ancient symbol of the UnderWorld guardian, the judge of the dead, and hunting packs of hounds play an important role in the Celtic religion and mythology. Just as Merlin is accompanied by an old wolf who was in the woods before him, so is another character in the *Vita* led to a ritualised death by chasing his hounds. The connection between wolf, dog and stag masks an initiatory sequence connected to hunting, which was clearly central to the Merlin tale, but is confused or deliberately underemphasised in Geoffrey's re-assembly of the material.[3]

The Winter Lament concludes with Merlin talking to his dying wolf; at this point we have the device of a listener overhearing the wild complaints and carrying news of Merlin to the messenger sent by Queen Ganeida, Merlin's sister and wife of King Rhydderch. The messenger finds Merlin 'on the very summit of a certain mountain', sitting by a fountain surrounded by hazel bushes and dense thorns.

This is our third *Image of Merlin* which, although almost an aside within the flow of the narrative, encapsulates certain key aspects of the native Celtic magical or spiritual traditions. Before examining this image, we should recap on those that have gone before:

1 Merlin as ruling King and leader of warriors, soon beset by grief;
2 Merlin as Wild Man in the woods, accompanied by a wolf;
3 Merlin sitting at the top of a mountain, by a spring surrounded with hazels and thorns, watching the animals run to and fro.

We could, without stretching the material too thinly, suggest that there is a simple topography in these images, one which is found in many medieval paintings and later alchemical or mystical illustrations:[4]

1 the city, and the plain of battle;
2 the woods, through which Merlin flees, possibly led by the wolf;
3 the sacred mountain topped by a spring (see Figure 3).

As Merlin progresses in his madness, he moves deeper into the aspects of Nature that directly represent his inner state. As we shall see, he does not proceed by straight lines, but by spirals and backward steps.

The spring or fountain surrounded by hazels is one of the primal images of the Celtic source of all being. The spring rises up from the mysterious depths, while the hazels fall into the spring to be used as food. In our present example, the spring is also guarded by thorns, another prime symbol of spiritual or magical potency, in which the source of power and life-giving energies is also protected from the presence of the unwise.[5]

This is Merlin's first encounter with the spring, but it is not his last. It is significant that at the spring, Merlin has his first cure, and is lured back to the settlements of mankind; his last cure is also effected by a magical spring, but only after a cycle of hardships and insights, plus a large chunk of acquired learning on the nature of the Worlds, the world, and of magical springs in general.

CHAPTER 4

I The question of the Four Seasons
II Lament for Guendoloena

Her eyes shone bright, as the stars at night, No diamonds could shine so.

Traditional folk song.

The messenger overhears Merlin ask one of the key magical questions, requesting an insight into the cycle of the seasons. Merlin longs for the new life of spring, and the messenger sings and plays to him, showing that Guendoloena (Merlin's abandoned wife) is indeed the essence of spring. The music is therapeutic, and Merlin returns to his senses.

THE QUESTION OF THE FOUR SEASONS

At last he saw Merlin . . . making his complaint in this manner,
    'O Thou who rulest all things, how does it happen that the seasons are not all the same, distinguished only by their four numbers? Now spring, according to its laws, provides flowers and leaves; summer gives crops, autumn ripe apples; icy winter follows and devours and wastes all the others, bringing rain and snow, and keeps them all away and harms with its tempests. And it does not permit the ground to produce variegated flowers, or the oak trees acorns, or the

apple trees dark red apples. O that there were no winter or white frost! That it were spring or summer, and that the cuckoo would come back singing, and the nightingale who softens sad hearts with her devoted song, and the turtle dove keeping her chaste vows, and that in new foliage other birds should sing in harmonious measures, delighting me with their music, while a new earth should breathe forth odors from new flowers under the green grass; that the fountains would also flow on every side with their gentle murmurs, and near by, under the leaves, the dove would pour forth her soothing laments and incite to slumber.

LAMENT FOR GUENDOLOENA

The messenger heard the prophet and broke off his lament with cadences on the cither he had brought with him that with it he might attract and soften the madman. Therefore making plaintive sounds with his fingers and striking the strings in order, he lay hidden behind him and sang in a low voice, 'O the dire groanings of mournful Guendoloena! O the wretched tears of weeping Guendoloena! I grieve for wretched dying Guendoloena! There was not among the Welsh a woman more beautiful than she. She surpassed in fairness the goddesses, and the petals of the privet, and the blooming roses and the fragrant lilies of the fields. The glory of spring shone in her alone, and she had the splendor of the stars in her two eyes, and splendid hair shining with the gleam of gold. All this has perished; all beauty has departed from her, both color and figure and also the glory of her snowy flesh. Now, worn out with much weeping, she is not what she was, for she does not know where the prince has gone, or whether he is alive or dead; therefore the wretched woman languishes and is totally wasted away through her long grief. With similar laments Ganieda weeps with her, and without consolation grieves for her lost brother. One weeps for her brother and the other for her husband, and both devote themselves to weeping and spend their time in sadness. No food nourishes them, nor does any sleep refresh them wandering at night through the brushwood, so great is the grief that consumes them both. Not otherwise did Sidonian Dido grieve when the ships had weighed anchor and Aeneas was in haste to depart; so most wretched Phyllis groaned and wept when Demophoon did not come back at the appointed time; thus Briseis wept for the absent Achilles. Thus the sister and the wife grieve together, and burn continually and completely with inward agonies.'

The messenger sang thus to his plaintive lyre, and with his music soothed the ears of the prophet that he might become more gentle and rejoice with the singer. Quickly the prophet arose and addressed the young man with pleasant words, and begged him to touch once more the strings with his fingers and to sing again his former song. The latter therefore set his fingers to the lyre and played over again the song that was asked for, and by his playing compelled the man, little by little, to put aside his madness, captivated by the sweetness of the lute.

THE QUESTION OF THE FOUR SEASONS

We now return to Merlin's questions regarding life, in the form of yet another sub-poem within the overall context of Geoffrey's verses. It is likely to be the conclusion of the Winter Lament, but raises an important question which will, in time, be answered by the bard Taliesin:[1] 'How does it happen that the seasons are not all the same?'

Merlin is revealing some progress on his path around the Wheel, for at the beginning of his lament he rails against winter, and his familiar wolf dies of starvation. At the end of this experience he has climbed the mystic mountain to the magical spring, but is not yet able to be cured by its waters. He does, however, ask the right question, which is 'What is the nature of the Wheel?'

Curiously his question is answered by his experiences immediately following the question, for he is soothed into a temporary sanity and returns to civilisation; the nature of the Wheel is that it goes around, and that we return from whence we began.

The messenger, sent by Merlin's sister, now practices one of the time-hallowed techniques of therapy: music. He plucks the cither or *crwth* and by its plaintive sounds attracts the madman's attention.

This scene is perhaps part of the progression of images, for if we set aside the literary context of the plot which holds the traditional poems together, we find the image of a madman or seer, driven wild by inner powers or overwhelming sorrow, being calmed by the power of music. This is an enduring concept, which has precedents at least as far back as *The Republic* of Plato, but is likely in the present case to be drawn from the Celtic traditions relating to the magical power of music.

The power of music

Music was anciently considered to be a physical expression of the properties of number and order, with the seven notes of the scale or mode corresponding to the Seven Planets. The use of music to calm Merlin, and so draw his attention to the lament for Guendoloena which follows, therefore gives us a clear image of the order of the cosmos being used to reattune the disorder of the deranged elemental psyche.

While we need this to be explained in some detail, it would have been a central item of general knowledge to the reasonably educated or traditionally orientated listener of the medieval period; such education came either through the Church and its inheritance of classical sources plus the influx of Arabic knowledge at the time, or from the traditional power ascribed to bards through long association with Celtic practices going back to the pre-Christian era.

Once again we find a suggestive sub-structure to the text, to the question and answer pattern which formed such a central part of oral techniques for communicating wisdom. Merlin has asked about the nature of the Seasons, and while this is later answered by a full exposition from the bard Taliesin, inspired by a goddess,[2] and is obviously reflected in Merlin's first return to civilisation, that same answer also comes to him immediately in the form of music.

As music was composed of the Four Elements and the Seven Spheres, the answer to Merlin's question 'What is the nature of the Wheel?' is physically manifested to him, though he does not consciously recognise it at the time.[3]

LAMENT FOR GUENDOLOENA

The power of music is employed by the messenger to liberate Merlin from his madness; there may be a remote suggestion of both classical and native mythology in this image, for messenger gods are connected to the invention of musical instruments (the lyre), and to the tricking or amusing of the aroused powerful gods (Hermes and Appollo).[4]

Once the prophet's attention has been gained, the messenger moves on to speak of his lamenting wife, Guendoloena. It is worth commenting at this stage that Merlin has not, in fact, made any prophecies during this early part of the story; he does not exhibit his powers of perception until he is tricked back to Rhydderch's court by the lament for his wife's and sister's grief.

The quality of this poem is interesting, as it seems more of a song or stylised structure than any other part of the *Vita*, except perhaps the lament for Rhydderch which follows in a later section and shares some of the symbolism. It is possible that Geoffrey has incorporated a well-known poem, and taken trouble to render it into Latin that parallels the Welsh or Breton original; as the poetic forms of the two cultures (Celtic and Roman) differ in many respects, it is to the imagery that we should go to find any connecting theme.

There are striking similarities between the description of Merlin's wife Guendoloena and traditional verses describing a native goddess; this theme is repeated in the *Mabinogion* with the magical creation of Blodeuedd the Flower Maiden. In Scots gaelic lore there are poems with similar symbolism, and it is likely that Geoffrey used an established form (which persisted in Celtic regions as late as the eighteenth century) or body of descriptive symbols which originally applied to a Flower Maiden or goddess of Spring and fertility.[5]

If we regard the imagery in this manner we immediately draw the relationship between Merlin as Wild Man at Winter, losing his totem or companion beast, living alone and bewailing the cold season, and Guendoloena at Spring, seeking to rejoin him.

> She surpassed in fairness the goddesses, and the petals of the
> privet, the blooming roses and the fragrant lilies of the field.
> The glory of spring shone in her alone, and she had the
> splendour of stars in her two eyes, and splendid hair shining
> with the gleam of gold.

The traditional use of maidens to symbolise divine feminine power was by no means suppressed during Geoffrey's time; it was soon to expand into the massive growth of literature relating to the Grail, and of course to the theme of courtly love. Merlin also employs some potent imagery in which a maiden changes shape, representing the goddess of the Land (in *The Prophecies*), and such images in verse, tale or song are likely to have been widespread in Geoffrey's circle of Norman-Celtic society.

More particularly, if Geoffrey is indeed drawing from the repertoire of itinerant or partly itinerant bards (a system of entertainment which persisted until the eighteenth century or later in Ireland, Brittany and Scotland in the form of harpers and reciters touring from house to house to entertain both gentry and common folk) he is reworking a symbolic theme that would have been presented in fragmented form via oral tradition.

This leads us to another subtlety in the overall structure of the *Vita Merlini*, for it fuses together elements which are likely to have been disparate in their traditional form: the remnants of a sophisticated system of symbolism well into decline despite its good state of oral preservation. It is Geoffrey who we have to thank for this fusion as it seems unlikely that he drew the connecting themes merely from his own imagination or from the work of his traditional sources alone.

The combination of traditional lore with the imaginative restructuring by a widely read and expressive poet (Geoffrey) gave the old Celtic magical themes a sudden boost into literary currency, something which they had not previously had. The effect upon resulting literature and culture worldwide need hardly be stated here, except to summarise that the direction and tone of much of English literature was set by *The History* and the *Vita*.

Guendoloena, therefore, is a type of goddess image, albeit disguised in the structure of the *Vita*. She is Merlin's neglected wife; the power of the Spring and rebirth to come, and at the same time the feminine principle which he has left behind in his fits of madness to live alone as a wild man.

We will find both of these themes to be closely related, and to be developed as the *Vita* progresses; Merlin allows his wife to remarry, as we shall see shortly, but kills her new husband. His feminine balance comes not from sexual union, which he outgrows as the poem progresses, but from the polarised companionship of his sister, who is also drawn into the messenger's grief poem towards the close. Superficially this change of sexual emphasis fits with the ethics of Christian virtue, but it masks a deeper and far-reaching spiritual and psychological understanding, exposition and experience.

With the introduction of Ganieda, both elements of Merlin's relationship to that which is female are stated, both mourning:

> One weeps for her brother and the other for her hus-
> band. . . . No food nourishes them, nor does any sleep
> refresh them wandering at night through the brushwood, so
> great is the grief that consumes them both.

Myths that relate to mourning for a lost lover are a basic element of ancient nature lore, but we should not take such themes as merely an indication of the seasonal cycle or the growth and decay of crops. The harmonic connection to the human psyche, to human relationships, and ultimately to the spiritual or deepest innermost polarities of the nature of being, are expressed by the simple sexual symbolism.

If we consider the images of this Lament, we find a raw power wasting in the woods (Merlin) with a lover waiting at spring (Merlin's sexual partner). Added to this, once the main theme of lamenting for lost love has been established, we find non-sensual feminine love (Merlin's sister) wandering thorny paths at night as an equal partner with the sensual lover. This imagery may be valuable in two ways. Firstly, the wife and sister were represented in ancient culture by two aspects of a female power, generally a triple goddess. This goddess was traditionally known as a Maiden, a Lover, and a Crone, representing three phases of female power in expression. Each of these in turn exercised certain magical powers with direct relationship to the development of human culture and to individual human consciousness. The polar relationship in the Merlin sequence is likely to be a remnant or restatement of this imagery.

The Maiden represented purity, unchanging wisdom, cultural development through use of the mind, and acted as the patroness of certain chosen men, heroes doomed to express and enact mythical and magical ventures for the benefit of the people.
The Lover represented the polarised sexual powers, fruitfulness, sensuality, fertility in the land, animals and humans.
The Crone represented death, breakdown, battle, and the mysterious powers of the UnderWorld which acted as the foundation for all life and manifestation.

Each of these three aspects of female divinity had in turn stellar parallels and mythical sequences which linked them to the passage of certain stars, planets, or configurations seen in the night sky at particular times of the year.

These elements each have a presence in the *Vita*, with the lover, the sister, and a mysterious woman who deals out madness and death, making appearances which are frequently interchanged. We should not expect or demand that the triplicity of ancient female power appears intact or in an archetypical mode, for this hardly ever occurs in early literature, or in tales and ballads which include the theme.

The connection between Merlin, star-lore, and a female power is clearly stated in *The Prophecies*, and in the later book of the *Vita* two reiterations occur. The most obvious is the literary repeat (with variations) of actual prophecies, which are clearly inserted as a type of corroborative evidence by Geoffrey, drawing upon the established popularity of his earlier presentation in *The History*. The second reiteration, however, is of more interest from the esoteric or psychological viewpoint, for it reaffirms the connections between Merlin's spiritual or inner growth and his relationship to specific aspects of feminine energy and consciousness; these in turn are linked to stellar observation and a type of astrological symbolism.

The fact that Merlin's sister is also the wife of King Rydderch, and displays resourcefulness in her adulterous love for another man, does not detract from the goddess theme, for the images and aspects merge into one another.[6] In other branches of the Merlin tradition his sister plays a slightly different role, and to grasp this fluid alteration of themes and polarities we must always remember that we are dealing with symbolism from a diffuse tradition, in which the primal magical images remain, but the religious or thematic rationalisations of pagan culture have been fragmented.

The second way in which the feminine characters are valuable is as direct emblems of the feminine aspects of the individual psyche. On a cultural or religious level they are shown as ancient goddesses, a powerful presentation which can interact with individual consciousness today, and is active in both revival paganism, the worship of the Virgin in Christian cults, and in primal religion worldwide. But the female polar powers are present in consciousness itself, and have been employed in meditation, visualisation, and transformative techniques for many centuries.[7]

The *Vita* is therefore a valid psychological document which relates the interaction between the polarised aspects of the psyche and leads towards their union through balance. Although many materialist psychologists would deny the effectiveness of mystical or religious lore remaining from both pagan and primal Christian sources, in esoteric psychology the magical images and powers merge smoothly with the personal psychic images or constructs. We can find this very process occurring repeatedly within the experiences of Merlin himself, and the conclusions which are drawn indirectly from his adventures.

Two classes of 'conclusion' are found in the *Vita*: those which directly express the results of Merlin's powers – his prophecies, his observations upon life, his final rejection of material society for a life of inner contemplation – and those which are inferred from the subtle symbolic progression from stage to stage, which is also a progression from state to state of awareness. It is this second class which holds the enduring magical themes drawn from both classical and Celtic tradition, although we tend to look for this type of material solely through its fragmented presence in the first class, where it is obvious, literary, and of less value as a coherent or effective system of inner growth.

Towards the close of the Lament for Guendoloena, Geoffrey brings in a number of classical sources – Dido and Aeneas, Phyllis and Demophoon, Briseis and Achilles – which are employed as stylish comparisons to round the sequence off, and are in keeping with the literary requirements of the period. The final sentence is worth comment: 'Thus the sister and the wife grieve together and burn continually and completely with inward agonies.' We have seen the pair tread thorny paths together, sleepless; now they burn with inward agonies. The classical allusions do not, in fact, meet up to the tone of the Celtic original and seem to be a required insertion. The image of both sister and wife burning inwardly is a clear statement of the unpolarised feminine or sexual energy (the actual physical gender being cyclical and irrelevant, as we are dealing with a mythical, transpersonal, and individual flow of related symbols).

There is perhaps another connection which may be drawn lightly here, one which occurs in other Merlin images or verses found in Geoffrey's reassemblies in both the *Vita* and *The*

History. Burning with grief, treading thorny paths, lamenting for lost love, all are images clearly stated in certain post-mortem traditions. This imagery is found in traditional verses linked to the UnderWorld, but is also part of worldwide metaphysics and mystical philosophy.

The holistic or harmonic nature of oral wisdom traditions is demonstrated very clearly by this poem; the Lament for Guendoloena combines a number of elements which are often falsely separated by the modern mind. No such dissection would have been required by Geoffrey's audience, and certainly not by the bardic sources with active currency of their songs and tales within the Celtic culture. Indeed, this poem could act as a model of the fertile cross-references that underpin and enrich an essentially oral tradition, whether we take it as superficial entertainment or at its deepest, most potent level. In a small community, songs and tales were constantly circulated not only at a 'professional' level in writing such as the chronicles or works of Geoffrey, or the declamations of the travelling story tellers, but also as an essential strand of the fabric of daily life. Pleasure, knowledge, and ultimately wisdom were all embodied in a constant stream of song, tale, or saying. It cannot be repeated too often or overemphasised that this is the ambience, the fertile earth, within which the *Vita* was both written out and heard by its listeners.

Many of the themes assembled by Geoffrey would be known to his audience, and many many lines of cross-reference are implied, underpinning the clearly stated comparisons such as the allusions to classical lovers pining for their partners. Within this web of relationships between themes or characters runs the core tradition from an earlier culture, in which transpersonal or transcendant wisdom is embodied in enduring images and tales of personal struggle with metaphysical or religious overtones, and occasional distinct stellar analogies.

Before moving on to our next motif, in which Merlin returns to human society for a while, it is worth summarising the elements of the Guendoloena poem in brief, as they run through the remainder of the *Vita* and are developed and resolved by Merlin's own spiritual growth:

1 Messenger uses the power of music to draw Merlin's attention to the neglected female elements within his life;

2 an image of feminine sexual and fertile beauty awaits him, one potential path of fulfilment;

3 an image of sisterly or non-sensual love also walks side by side with the fertile beauty; they are each aspects of a powerful image of the Triple Goddess widespread in pagan cultures;

4 the cycle of the Seasons is implied, with Merlin at Winter and his lover at Spring;

5 there is some implication of the mysterious paths of the Otherworld and the ancient instructions to the soul which act as guidance after physical death;

6 a stellar or astrological relationship is not yet stated, but will be found in later sections which resolve the cycles of polarity found here, referring back to the image of the lover and the sister upon a higher or transpersonal level.

CHAPTER 5

I Merlin's first return
II The Threefold Death: 1
III The Threefold Death: 2

Mortality shall return . . . the camp of Venus shall be
restored, nor shall the arrows of Cupid cease to wound; the
fountain of a river shall be turned to blood, and two kings
shall fight a duel.

The Prophecies of Merlin.

Merlin is cured by the power of music, and returns to the court of
King Rhydderch to rejoin his wife and sister. He cannot endure the
presence of crowds of people, and seeks to flee. He is restrained and
given further musical therapy, and yet he refuses the most tempting
bribes from the king. He is bound with a strong chain, and
refuses to speak or laugh; Merlin and Rhydderch are in conflict.

But something makes him smile at last, and further bribes
will not encourage him to reveal the cause. Finally he is granted
his freedom as reward for revelation; he states that his sister
has deceived the king her husband with another man. Ganieda
tests his sanity by presenting a youth in three different
disguises, and Merlin predicts a different death for each
presentation. He is set free, but presumed mad. But in years to
come, his triple prophecy comes true in a most surprising manner.

MERLIN'S FIRST RETURN

So Merlin became mindful of himself, and he recalled what

he used to be, and he wondered at his madness and he hated it. His former mind returned and his sense came back to him, and, moved by affection, he groaned at the names of his sister and of his wife, since his mind was now restored to him, and he asked to be led to the court of King Rhydderch. The other obeyed him, and straightway they left the woods and came, rejoicing together, to the city of the king. So the queen was delighted by regaining her brother and the wife became glad over the return of her husband. They vied with each other in kissing him and they twined their arms about his neck, so great was the affection that moved them. The king also received him with such honor as was fitting, and the chieftains who thronged the palace rejoiced in the city.

But when Merlin saw such great crowds of men present he was not able to endure them; he went mad again, and, filled anew with fury, he wanted to go to the woods, and he tried to get away by stealth. Then Rhydderch ordered him to be restrained and a guard posted over him, and his madness to be softened with the cither; and he stood about him grieving, and with imploring words begged the man to be sensible and to stay with him, and not to long for the grove or to live like a wild beast, or to want to abide under the trees when he might hold a royal scepter and rule over a warlike people. After that he promised that he would give him many gifts, and he ordered people to bring him clothing and birds, dogs and swift horses, gold and shining gems, and cups that Wayland had engraved in the city of Segontium.[1] Every one of these things Rhydderch offered to the prophet and urged him to stay with him and leave the woods.

The prophet rejected these gifts, saying, 'Let the dukes who are troubled by their own poverty have these, they who are not satisfied with a moderate amount but desire a great deal. To these gifts I prefer the groves and broad oaks of Calidon, and the lofty mountains with green pastures at their feet. Those are the things that please me, not these of yours – take these away with you, King Rhydderch. My Calidonian forest rich in nuts, the forest that I prefer to everything else, shall have me.'

Finally since the king could not retain the sad man by any gifts, he ordered him to be bound with a strong chain lest, if free, he might seek the deserted groves. The prophet, when he felt the chains around him and he could not go as a free man to the Calidonian forests, straightway fell to grieving and remained sad and silent, and took all joy from his face so that he did not utter a word or smile.[2]

Meanwhile the queen was going through the hall looking for the king, and he, as was proper, greeted her as she came and took her by the hand and bade her sit down, and, embracing her, pressed her lips in a kiss. In so doing he turned his face toward her and saw a leaf hanging in her hair; he reached out his fingers, took it and threw it on the ground, and jested joyfully with the woman he loved. The prophet turned his eyes in that direction and smiled, and made the men standing about look at him in wonder since he was not in the habit of smiling. The king too wondered and urged the madman to tell the cause of his sudden laugh, and he added to his words many gifts. The other was silent and put off explaining his laugh. But more and more Rhydderch continued to urge him with riches and with entreaties until at length the prophet, vexed at him, said in return for his gift, 'A miser loves a gift and a greedy man labors to get one; these are easily corrupted by gifts and bend their minds in any direction they are bidden to. What they have is not enough for them, but for me the acorns of pleasant Calidon and the shining fountains flowing through fragrant meadows are sufficient. I am not attracted by gifts; let the miser take his, and unless liberty is given me and I go back to the green woodland valleys I shall refuse to explain my laughter.'

Therefore when Rhydderch found that he could not influence the prophet by any gift, and he could not find out the reason for the laughter, straightway he ordered the chains to be loosed and gave him permission to seek the deserted groves, that he might be willing to give the desired explanation. Then Merlin, rejoicing that he could go, said,

'This is the reason I laughed, Rhydderch. You were by a single act both praiseworthy and blameworthy. When just now you removed the leaf that the queen had in her hair without knowing it, you acted more faithfully toward her than she did toward you when she went under the bush where her lover met her and lay with her; and while she was lying there supine with her hair spread out, by chance there caught in it the leaf that you, not knowing all this, removed.'

MERLIN'S FIRST RETURN

We have followed the prophet through a journey that is physical, psychological and metaphysical; his progress through the outer landscape of Wales is directly attuned to his progress through an inner landscape of spiritual growth, a maturity which he cannot gain without a third level, that in which the psyche is attuned to images of potent divinity expressing themes of polarity. This level is in turn interwoven with an ancient astrological or stellar lore, which is explicitly stated in *The Prophecies* and given a gradual unfolding in the *Vita*.

It is not until Merlin has endured a number of hardships and made a series of realisations that we find the prophetic and stellar lore appearing in an open manner. This development of the text is a statement of Merlin's own development, and is suggestive of the traditional (probably Druidic) origins of the cycle of wisdom poems which Geoffrey reassembled. We are then able, retrospectively, to look back and realise that these magical themes were present continually from the very beginning, in which Merlin initially acts as a seasonal stereotype without true spiritual consciousness. He dances back and forth, a dance in which the Wheel of the earthly life is a reflection of the Wheel of stellar life. This will become much clearer as we proceed with his tale.

The powerful therapy of music reminds Merlin of his lost female partner, and his intellectual clarity is reawakened. His first act is to *consciously* request further music from the messenger; he is now awakened from the semi-dream of nature

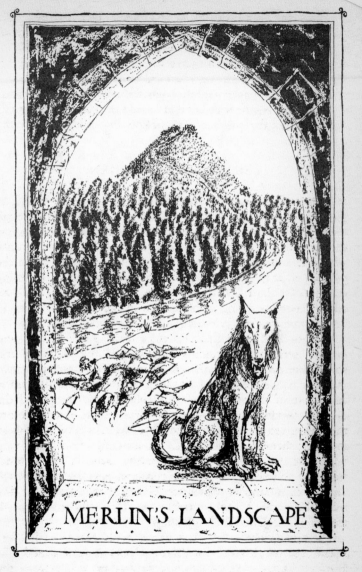

Figure 3 *Merlin's landscape*

and uses his own will to heal himself. In this sense the messenger (Mercury or Hermes in classical symbolism) is Merlin's own intellect, and this use of the messenger is found in other traditional British sources, where an equally important role is played.[3]

'So Merlin became mindful of himself, and he recalled what he used to be, and he wondered at his madness and he hated it.' Merlin is about to make his first return to human society, his first spiralling step backwards in his cyclical progression. This spiral is shown in our Figure 2, a modern form of the Wheel of Life and Change which was central to the education of the ancient Mysteries.

The Wheel, shown in Celtic Christian context as the equal-armed cross with its associated traceries, is a very ancient symbol indeed, not limited to solar or seasonal meaning, but embracing such meaning within an open-ended cycle of symbols.

Merlin has travelled thus: from the throne to the plain of battle; from the plain of battle to the wildwood; from the wildwood to the spring at the mountain top; now he goes from the mountain top back to the plain, and enters the city of King Rhydderch (see Figure 4).

Man leaves his own ruling outer consciousness, reverts to primal untuned nature, which propels him to the source of life and energy. There his relationship to feminine principles is brought back into his awareness through a rejuvenation of his intellect, set in order by music (the power of the Muse), a reflection of the solar and planetary order which he is soon to perceive as a stellar seer.

This reharmonised consciousness leads him to the court of the king; now the ruling quality is exteriorised by the figure of Rhydderch, acting as a power of rulership which Merlin has grown beyond in his transformative madness, but which he has not fully left behind. It is significant that it is during Merlin's first return that he exhibits his first supernormal perception.

The use of Merlin's seership seems at first trivial; he discovers his sister to be unfaithful to her husband the king. But in our magical context of polarity, and the mystical theme of

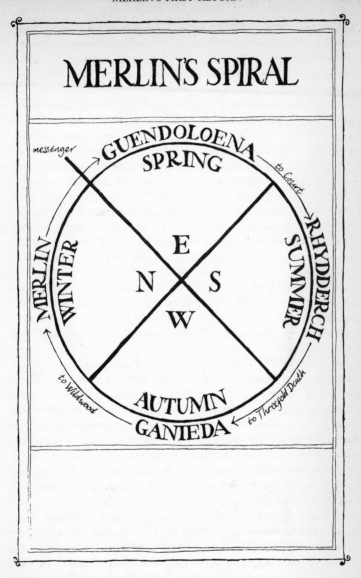

Figure 4 *Merlin's spiral*

spiritual growth through a dance or journey in which inner dimensions are linked to both microcosm and macrocosm, this appearance of seership with the relationship between sister and king is extremely important.

The figure of the king is no longer paramount, his rulership is already diminished (Merlin has rejected his own kingship as ruler of a powerful clan and chosen madness and the wildwood); so Merlin's relative by marriage is shown as a cuckold ... the feminine principle is not subservient to the male stereotype. We could express this more traditionally and poetically and state that the goddess is already active in the tale, changing her allegiance as she wills; this change is intimately linked to Merlin's power of seership, and to a most potent image of sacrifice which follows hard upon his first exhibition of far-knowledge, the image of the Threefold Death.

But we are anticipating the sequence of events, and Merlin first exhibits an anti-reaction to the city life, to the ordinary outward world. In the midst of the general rejoicing at his return, Merlin is oppressed by the great throng of people, and his madness begins afresh. He seeks the woods, tries to creep away, but is restrained forcibly, and given further musical therapy!

This reaction is typical of the first return, and is known to mystical techniques, magical training, and in religious devotion. Once the inner life and divine consciousness have been experienced, however briefly or incoherently, the return to the outer world is difficult; there is a conflict, a longing to flee, yet the knowledge that the individual must stay and respond to human requirements. Merlin's behaviour is typical of seers, prophets, mystics and visionaries worldwide, and also reveals a psychic phenomenon upon the mystical path during the early stages of development.

This conflict is stated in the conversation between King Rhydderch and Merlin; under guard, soothed by music, the wild man is begged, bribed, and coerced to remain in the company of regular human society. The king 'begged the man to be sensible ... when he might hold a royal scepter and rule over a warlike people. After that he promised that he would give him many gifts. . . .' The Biblical parallel would not have been lost upon Geoffrey's audience; just as the prophet Merlin is tempted by the lure of the world, so was the saviour Jesus tempted. There is a strong implication that Merlin is the Celtic equivalent of Jesus, with the *Vita* acting in relationship to *The History* just as the New Testament acts in relationship to the Old. Such a connection should not be drawn too tightly, but the harmonic link is present, and in early Western culture Merlin was often linked with Jesus as a prophet, a tendency which was gradually supressed by the Roman Church.[4]

There is no suggestion here that Merlin is equal to or a replacement for Jesus in the Western religious or mystical consciousness; both Merlin and the historical Jesus were prophets within their own native traditions; the difference lies in the degree of Divine origin or realisation, which is a matter of religion and not of mythology or psychology or even of magical exposition. We must attempt to grasp that during the early centuries of Celtic Christianity predating the power-play of the political Roman Church, there was a vast sophisticated mythology from pagan culture interwoven with the infant faith of the new religion. The ambience of this situation persisted within the oral traditions until very late indeed, and is still found even in the twentieth century in folk ballads and tales where pagan and Christian symbolism are innocently and harmonically merged together without any discomfort, dogmatic argument, or diminution of basic Christian faith.[5]

Merlin, meanwhile, is being tempted to remain in the world; Rhydderch orders people '. . . to bring him clothing and birds, dogs and swift horses, gold and shining gems, and cups that Wayland had engraved in the city of Segontium'. All the benefits, in fact, of the princely material life which led in the first instance to the battle and to Merlin's grief and madness. This much of the Wheel, at least, he has become aware of: that material benefits turn to despair, they are a temporal illusion. 'Let the dukes who are troubled by their own poverty have these. . . . My Calidonian forest, rich in nuts, shall have me.'

But the world is not easily rejected, and a mere statement of rejection is not sufficient; indeed, it causes the prophet to be enchained by the king. We find another perceptive truth here: the attempt to be 'free' leads directly to a greater slavery. The outward-seeking flow of consciousness is not merely turned around by resistance, it will fight back by persuasion and finally by rigidity and imprisonment until the correct paths to resolution and liberation are found.

Our next image of Merlin is that he is chained, in gloom and despair, longing to be free, but unable to leave the court of the king. This despair is symbolised in various ways in mystical traditions, and has its counterpart in everyday consciousness which we can all recognise and identify with.

The way to liberation, however, is mysterious, and we now enter upon a motif which is directly pertinent to the theme of mystical development and the growth of the elemental psyche.

Merlin laughs as the king brushes a leaf, lovingly, from his wife's hair. Intrigued by this sudden mirth in the midst of such despair, the king questions the mad seer, offering him further and greater gifts if he will only tell the cause of his change of mood. 'Let the miser take his [gifts], and unless liberty is given me . . . I shall refuse to explain my laughter.'

So Merlin is unchained, given permission to leave in exchange for the tantalising reasons for his mirth. He explains that his sister has been unfaithful to the king, and the leaf so lovingly brushed away had come into her hair while lying with her lover.

The development of this motif is complex, and Geoffrey or his source has cunningly worked a number of levels and themes into it. Before taking the story any further, we should note that it is the apparently *sexual* antics of his sister, her cuckolding of the king (in old-fashioned terminology) that leads directly to Merlin's freedom; it is also the subject of his first display of seership. The incident is by no means as trivial as it might appear, and is certainly not just an entertaining insertion into the legend from an exotic source.[6]

We use the term 'cuckolding' very deliberately, as it reappears in a later motif where Merlin is betrayed by *his* wife and uses a set of horns, the traditional symbol applied to the cuckold for reasons not exclusively superficially phallic, to kill his rival. This group of symbols will be dealt with in its proper place.

Ganieda is not dismissed by the narrator as a faithless wife, and there is no moral retribution attached to her behaviour other than by her husband. Indeed, she goes on to demonstrate her skill in deception, as it seems, and so introduces an extremely ancient sacrificial motif into the tale, one which is central to the development of Merlin's inner awareness, yet is offered to us as a sub-plot within the main tale.

THE THREEFOLD DEATH: 1

Rhydderch suddenly became sad at this accusation and turned his face from her and cursed the day he had married her. But she, not at all moved, hid her shame behind a smiling face and said to her husband, 'Why are you sad, my love? Why do you become so angry over this thing and blame me unjustly, and believe a madman who, lacking sound sense, mixes lies with the truth? The man who believes him becomes many times more a fool than he is. Now then, watch, and if I am not mistaken I will show you that he is crazy and has not spoken the truth.'

There was in the hall a certain boy, one of many, and the ingenious woman catching sight of him straightway thought of a novel trick by which she might convict her brother of falsehood. So she ordered the boy to come in and asked her brother to predict by what death the lad should die. He answered, 'Dearest sister, he shall die, when a man, by falling from a high rock.' Smiling at these words, she ordered the boy to go away and take off the clothes he was wearing and put on others and to cut off his long hair; she bade him come back to them thus that he might seem to them a different person. The boy obeyed her, for he came back to them with his clothes changed as he had been ordered to do. Soon the queen asked her brother again, 'Tell your dear sister what the death of this boy will be like.' Merlin answered, 'This boy when he grows up shall, while out of his mind, meet with a violent death in a tree.' When he had finished she said to her husband, 'Could this false prophet lead you so far astray as to make you believe that I had committed so great a crime? And if you will notice with how much sense he has spoken this about the boy, you will believe that the things he said about me were made up so that he might get away to the woods. Far be it from me to do such a thing! I shall keep my bed chaste, and chaste shall I always be while the breath of life is in me. I convicted him of falsehood when I asked him about the death of the boy. Now I shall do it again; pay attention and judge.'

When she had said this she told the boy in an aside to go out and put on woman's clothing, and to come back thus. Soon the boy left and did as he was bid, for he came back in woman's clothes just as though he were a woman, and he stood in front of Merlin to whom the queen said banteringly, 'Say brother, tell me about the death of this girl.' 'Girl or not she shall die in the river,' said her brother to her, which made King Rhydderch laugh at his reasoning; since when asked about the death of a single boy Merlin had predicted three different kinds. Therefore Rhydderch thought he had spoken falsely about the queen, and did not believe him, but grieved, and hated the fact that he had trusted him and had condemned his beloved. The queen, seeing this, forgave him and kissed and caressed him and made him joyful.

THE THREEFOLD DEATH: 2

Guendoloena remained sadly in the door watching him and so did the queen, both moved by what had happened to their friend, and they marveled that a madman should be so familiar with secret things and should have known of the love affair of his sister. Nevertheless they thought that he lied about the death of the boy since he told of three different deaths when he should have told of one. Therefore his speech seemed for long years to be an empty one until the time when the boy grew to manhood; then it was made apparent to all and convincing to many. For while he was hunting with his dogs he caught sight of a stag hiding in a grove of trees; he loosed the dogs who, as soon as they saw the stag, climbed through unfrequented ways and filled the air with their baying. He urged on his horse with his spurs and followed after, and urged on the huntsmen, directing them, now with his horn and now with his voice, and he bade them go more quickly. There was a high mountain surrounded on all sides by rocks with a stream flowing through the plain at its foot; thither the animal fled until he came to the river, seeking a hiding place after the unusual manner of its kind. The young man pressed on and passed straight over the mountain, hunting for the stag among the rocks lying about. Meanwhile it happened, while his impetuosity was leading him on, that his horse slipped from a high rock and the man fell over a precipice into the river, but so that one of his feet caught in a tree, and the rest of his body was submerged in the stream. Thus he fell, and was drowned, and hung from a tree, and by this threefold death made the prophet a true one.

THE THREEFOLD DEATH: 1

Before examining the first prophecy expressed in the *Vita*, that of the Threefold Death, we should be aware that in other tales it is the prophet himself who suffers this death; it is his prediction for the ending of his own life.[7]

In the *Vita*, however, the prediction is shunted onto a minor character in the context of Ganieda's unfaithfulness to her husband. The imagery remains true to the original theme which is found in Celtic or British mythology in several sources. The separation from Merlin himself makes a rather odd ending to the overall story of the *Vita*, for as we shall see, the prophetic spirit passes from him and enters his sister at the close of the poem.

We can regard this removal of the Threefold Death from Merlin in two possible ways, which are related in concept. Firstly, it may simply have been too suggestive of pagan lore, and creates once again the parallel between Merlin and Jesus, as both suffered a curious sacrificial death. Secondly, Geoffrey seeks an elegant and philosophical ending to his poem, in which the characters of Merlin, Ganieda, and Taliesin retire to the woods together. In one sense this represents not merely a weakening of the older Celtic theme, but a removal of its magical elements to a higher level, a transformation which retains the pagan elements but gives them an acceptable and spiritual ending in keeping with medieval Christianity.[8] We should not push this point too far, for the *Vita Merlini* is first and last a pagan cycle of mysteries and magic. There are very few overtly Christian terms or concepts, and even in the case of the Threefold Death, the motif itself is not done away with; it is thinly disguised by its attachment to a youth in Rhydderch's court.

If the *Vita* is intimately concerned with polarities of energy and consciousness expressed in the only symbolic language available through the oral wisdom traditions of the West, then the sub-textual elements of Merlin's relationship with his sister, and the parallels between Ganieda's unfaithfulness and the remarrying of Guendoloena, Merlin's wife, offer many suggestive insights into the human powers of transformation through imagery. Indeed, reducing the images of the scene at Rhydderch's court to very basic units, we find the following:

1 a King sitting at his court;
2 a wild man chained in his presence;
3 a woman who orders the appearance of (a) a boy, (b) a boy in disguise, (c) a boy dressed as a woman.

These are the elements of ritual drama; they may be found in attenuated but clearly related forms in folk dramas or mummer's plays into the twentieth century, and in a small number of traditional dance-drama ceremonies attached to seasonal festivals.[9]

Not only has the Threefold Death been removed from the immediate relationship to Merlin, but it has been incorporated into a scene which would have been well known to Geoffrey's audience in various forms, the life-death-resurrection drama found in folklore worldwide. Such dramas would have formed part of traditional entertainments of any household or community, and would have been linked to Celtic festivals, such as the rising and setting of the Pleiades in May and November.[10] The sequence would have been not only familiar to the audience but filled with implications of the customary rituals, probably divorced from any conscious magical or religious attributes but still potent in the communal imagination and still essential to the rhythm of agricultural life.

On a more archetypical level, we could refer the basic images listed above to a divine or mythological source: the king represents justice or rule; the prophet represents the wild powers of nature and the unpredictable raw energies of life; the boy represents the many aspects of human incarnation or polarity, but also is chosen as a sacrificial victim to combine all such aspects into one; the queen represents the goddess who directs all the drama from her originative position of power.

Between the rule of balance and the wild forces of nature, humankind enacts many changing roles; in certain individuals these roles are concentrated and combined into one sacrificial act that accelerates the cycles of the Wheel of Life or cuts across them. Such powerful sacrifices are directed by the goddess. The implications are complex but not difficult; such magical or metaphysical matters work through harmonic relationship rather than through direct cause and effect.

Returning to the thread of the narrative, we find that Merlin's prediction of three separate deaths (falling, hanging, drowning) is used as proof that he cannot predict accurately, and therefore that he is wrong in his revelation concerning the queen. There follows a short interlude in which Ganieda pleads for the case of Merlin's wife who is about to be neglected yet again. We shall pass over this, and return to it after we have dealt with the Threefold Death. The insertion of a further section of the Guendoloena relationship is a subtlety from Geoffrey; he has split the traditional themes up and intermixed their resolution for dramatic effect.

Merlin's three predictions are worth repeating precisely as they have direct bearing upon the sacrificial theme, the madness theme, and, as we shall shortly discover, the theme of a magical hunt:

1 'he shall die, when a man, by falling from a high rock';
2 'when he grows up he shall, while out of his mind, meet with a violent death in a tree';
3 'girl or not she shall die in the river'.

THE THREEFOLD DEATH: 2

Therefore his speech seemed for long years to be an empty one until the time when the boy came to manhood; then it was apparent to all and convincing to many.

Through the contrivance and dramatic effect of Geoffrey, the conclusion to the Threefold Death prophecy comes after we have been introduced to a new theme of remarriage, in which Merlin frees his wife from her marriage bonds, or seems to do so.[11]

The image of the boy's unusual fate is very clearly stated by Geoffrey, and may be summarised as follows:

A young man falls over a precipice; one of his feet is caught in a tree; he drowns while hanging upside down with his body partly submerged (see Figure 5).

This is an ancient and effective magical image, shown for several centuries through the Tarot trump, the Hanged Man. The *Vita* pre-dates the appearance of Tarot images by at least two centuries, and is one of the earliest sources of such imagery in connection with a wisdom tale or metaphysical text.

The meaning ascribed to the Tarot card, the Hanged Man, is identical to that found in the ancient tales: sacrifice in connection to higher ends beyond the mere individuality. This is not identical to and should not be confused with martyrdom or humility in the Christian sense of bowing to authority and suffering thereby. A.E. Waite, writing in 1910, described the Hanged Man thus:

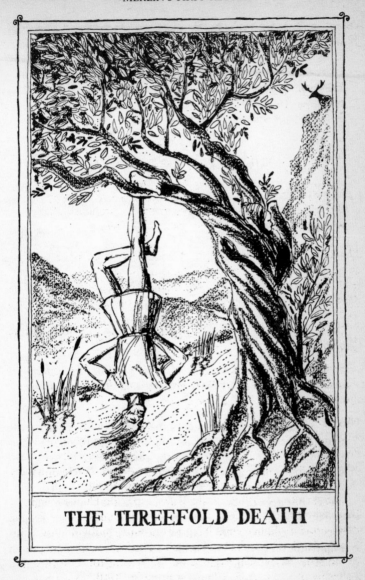

THE THREEFOLD DEATH

Figure 5 *The Threefold Death*

The gallows from which he is suspended forms a *Tau* cross, while the figure, from the position of the legs, forms a fylfot cross. There is a nimbus about the head. . . . It should be noted that (1) the tree of sacrifice is living wood, with leaves thereon; (2) that the face expresses deep entrancement, not suffering; (3) that the figure as a whole suggests life in suspension, but life and not death.

Waite describes a Tarot image redesigned to a certain extent by himself, but drawn directly from the anonymous traditional cards which permeated Europe during the early Renaissance. The similarity to the image in the *Vita* written out during the twelfth century is striking.[12]

The Threefold Death image employed by Geoffrey has obvious connections to the Christian crucifixion, but a different cultural background. An early Celtic inscription and image shows a man hanging from a tree, and the name ESUS. This predates the Christian event, and is one of a number of hanged god images which include the Norse Odin, the Celtic Esus, the Christian Jesus, the Hanged Man of the Tarot, and of course the Threefold Death image in the *Vita Merlini*.[13]

In our Appendix 7, the metaphysical and magical symbols of the image are discussed in detail; at this point in the examination of the main narrative we need to be aware of the image as follows:

1 A predicted triple death, culminating in an image that has endured through pictoral tradition in magic, proto-psychology and metaphysics to the present day.

2 The image is connected to a primal drama in which disparate sexual roles are unified in a chosen individual who meets the triple death.

3 The imagery is closely connected to the cycle of the Four Elements, described at length by the bard Taliesin in an important set of teachings which follow later in the main narrative. This Elemental theme is described in Appendix VII.

4 The Elemental cycle is inseparable from the old magical

Seasonal cycle; in this sense the Hanged One represents a synthesis of Merlin's spiralling journey around the primal year and the modes of consciousness associated with such a journey.

5 The Threefold Death is directly linked to Merlin himself in variants of the tale; it is a concentrated form of the expanded spiritual journey found throughout the *Vita Merlini*.

There are two further aspects which connect harmonically to both Tarot images and to Merlin's own period as a wild man of the woods.

1 The young man falls over a cliff to meet his triple death. In some Tarot images, the Fool, another major trump, appears to be about to step unwittingly over a cliff. He, like Merlin, is led by a totem canine beast, in this case a dog.[14] The image of falling over a cliff is embedded in the psyche as one of plunging into the unknown, and connects to a series of tales, magical instructions, and parables revealing the operations of inner spiritual growth.

2 The young man is 'out of his mind', inflamed by the passions of the hunt. The pursuit of the stag into the mountains is described in detail in the *Vita* and sets the imaginative scene for the Threefold Death. We shall shortly find that Merlin becomes Lord of the Animals, leading a herd of stags and goats, while riding upon a great stag. Merlin, in his wildwood phase, is connected to the stag and therefore to the hunt that leads to sacrificial death. In Celtic myth, the souls of the dead are pursued across the sky by a Wild Hunt led by the god of death and the UnderWorld.[15]

The Wild Hunt is associated with the festival of Hallowe'en, at which time the spirits of the dead are said to be close to the world of the living, and the gates between the worlds open wide. There is a very specific line of connection in this symbolism which plays a part in the Merlin theme and his link to the Threefold Death. Before moving on to the theme of marital freedom, this last symbolic resonance must be explored.

Hallowe'en is derived from a Celtic festival, Samhain. This in turn is derived from a ritual festival known worldwide and connected to passage of the Pleiades through the year. The polar opposite festival (Beltane) occurs around the beginning of May. The rising and setting of the Pleiades marked vital turning points of the year.[16]

In Merlin's *Prophecies*, the Pleiades and Orion, who is mythologically associated with the Pleiades due to their apparent positions in the night sky, play an important role. They mark the turning points of a metaphysical journey inseparably linked to their physical role as guiding constellations to travellers upon the sea. On a deeper level they act as matrices or mediators for cosmic powers which are graphically described by Merlin in his apocalyptic Vision.[17]

Hallowe'en, as we have said, is traditionally connected to the passage of the Wild Hunt, to a primal Hunter deity (closely linked to the image of Orion) who is also a woodland power, Lord of the Animals. He is very similar to the role taken by Merlin in the early parts of the *Vita*. But the connections reach further than this.

In the parallel tales of Lailoken, from Scots tradition, the prophet is 'given over to the angels of Satan,' and until his dying day is cursed to have 'communion with the creatures of the wood'. Lailoken, who predicts the Threefold Death for himself, is saved by Saint Kentigern, who challenges him and asks if he was ever a Christian and believed in God, and then demands how he came into the wildwood in the first place. This has striking connections to the old Scottish ballad of *Tam Lin* in which a knight is ensnared by the Fairy Queen of the wood, and a maiden first challenges his Christianity and mortality, to assert that he is indeed worth saving, then saves him by a series of magical transformations. Tam Lin undergoes these changes at Hallowe'en, and such shape changing plays a central role in *The Prophecies of Merlin*. The fairies have taken the usual confused place of the 'angels of Satan', for both Fairies and Otherworld Daemons were associated inaccurately with evil by the Church that sought to rid itself of the pagan practices.

We find this type of symbolism taken up in the Scottish

ballad and romance of *Thomas the Rhymer*, who is also carried off to the Otherworld by the Fairy Queen, who shows him a tree with poisoned magical fruit, and confers upon him the gift of prophecy. This tree appears in the *Vita Merlini* at the crucial scene of Merlin's final cure from wildwood madness.[18]

Clearly we are encountering not a series of derivative fragments but expressions of a very coherent magical transformative tradition. We shall return to some of these themes repeatedly as they are expressed in the main narrative.

CHAPTER 6
I Merlin and Guendoloena
II First star-lore
III Lord of the Animals

Virgo shall mount upon the back of Sagittarius, and darken her maiden flowers.

The Prophecies of Merlin.

Merlin tries to return to the woods, but his wife and sister seek to stop him. He is forced to make a decision about his wife; should she or should she not remarry? He releases her, but with a curious veiled threat. During the years that follow, she remarries.

Coherent observation of the night skies reveals to Merlin that political changes have arisen, and that Guendoloena has taken another husband. He mounts upon a stag, and with a herd of stags, deer and she-goats, attends the wedding place. His gift turns out to be a strange and violent death for the bridegroom.

MERLIN AND GUENDOLOENA

Meanwhile Merlin planned to go to the woods, and he left his dwelling and ordered the gates to be opened; but his sister stood in his way and with rising tears begged him to remain with her for a while and to put aside his madness. The hard-hearted man would not desist from his project but kept trying to open the doors, and he strove to leave and raged and fought and by his clamor forced the servants to open. At length, since no one could hold him back when he wanted to go, the queen quickly ordered Guendoloena, who was absent, to come to make him desist. She came and on her knees begged him to remain; but he spurned her prayers and would not stay, nor would he, as he was accustomed to do, look upon her with a joyful face. She grieved and dissolved in tears and tore her hair, and scratched her cheeks with her nails and rolled on the ground as though dying. The queen seeing this said to him, 'This Guendoloena who is dying thus for you, what shall she do? Shall she marry again or do you bid her remain a widow, or go with you wherever you are going? For she will go, and with you she will joyfully inhabit the groves and the green woodland meadows provided she has your love.' To this the prophet answered, 'Sister I do not want a cow that pours out water in a broad fountain like the urn of the Virgin in summer-time, nor shall I change my care as Orpheus once did when Eurydice gave her baskets to the boys to hold before she swam back across the Stygian sands. Freed from both of you I shall remain without the taint of love. Let her therefore be given a proper opportunity to marry and let him whom she shall choose have her. But let the man who marries her be careful that he never gets in my way or comes near me; let him keep away for fear lest if I happen to meet him he may feel my flashing sword. But when the day of the solemn wedding comes and the different viands are distributed to the guests, I shall be present in person, furnished with seemly gifts, and I shall profusely endow Guendoloena when she is given away.' When he had finished he said farewell to each of them and went away, and with no one to hinder him he went back to the woods he longed for . . . living like a wild beast, subsisting on frozen moss, in the snow, in the rain, in the cruel blasts of the wind. And this pleased him more than administering laws throughout his cities and ruling over fierce people. Meanwhile Guendoloena, since her husband was leading a life like this with his woodland flock through

the passing years, was married in accordance with her
husband's permission.

MERLIN'S FIRST SIGN OF STAR-LORE

It was night and the horns of the bright moon were shining,
and all the lights of the vault of heaven were gleaming; the
air was clearer than usual, for cruel, frigid Boreas had driven
away the clouds and had made the sky serene again and had
dried up the mists with his arid breath. From the top of a
lofty mountain the prophet was regarding the courses of the
stars, speaking to himself out in the open air. 'What does this
ray of Mars mean? Does its fresh redness mean that one king
is dead and that there shall be another? So I see it, for
Constantine has died and his nephew Conan, through an evil
fate and the murder of his uncle, has taken the crown and is
king. And you, highest Venus, who slipping along within
your ordered limits beneath the zodiac are accompanying the
sun in his course, what about this double ray of yours that is
cleaving the air? Does not its division indicate a severing of
my love? Such a ray indeed shows that loves are divided.
Perhaps Guendoloena has left me in my absence and now
clings to another man and rejoices in his embraces. So I lose;
so another enjoys her. So my rights are taken away from me
while I dally. So it is surely, for a slothful lover is beaten by
one who is not slothful or absent but is right on hand. But I
am not jealous; let her marry now under favorable auspices
and let her enjoy her new husband with my permission. And
when to-morrow's sun shall shine I will go and take with me
the gift I promised her when I left.'

MERLIN AS LORD OF THE ANIMALS

So he spoke and went about all the woods and groves and
collected a herd of stags in a single line, and the deer and she-
goats likewise, and he himself mounted a stag. And when day
dawned he came quickly, driving the line before him to the

place where Guendoloena was to be married. When he arrived he forced the stags to stand patiently outside the gates while he cried aloud, 'Guendoloena! Guendoloena! Come! Your presents are looking for you!' Guendoloena therefore came quickly, smiling and marvelling that the man was riding on the stag and that it obeyed him, and that he could get together so large a number of animals and drive them before him just as a shepherd does the sheep that he is in the habit of driving to the pastures.

The bridegroom stood watching from a lofty window and marvelling at the rider on his seat, and he laughed. But when the prophet saw him and understood who he was, at once he wrenched the horns from the stag he was riding and shook them and threw them at the man and completely smashed his head in, and killed him and drove out his life into the air. With a quick blow of his heels he set the stag to flying and was on his way back to the woods. At these happenings the servants rushed out from all sides and quickly followed the prophet through the fields. But he ran ahead so fast that he would have reached the woods untouched if a river had not been in his way; but while his beast was hurriedly leaping over the torrent Merlin slipped from his back and fell into the rapid waves. The servants lined the shore and captured him as he swam, and bound him and took him home and gave him to his sister.

MERLIN AND GUENDOLOENA

Merlin now seeks to return to the wildwood; his true prophecy has been made to appear false, but the entire drama has masked a deeper meaning. We have the image of Merlin raging at the gates of the city, striving to escape, while his sister reasons with him, striving to bring him to his senses. It is noteworthy that she does not blame him in any way for revealing her unfaithfulness, a matter which is immediately passed over as we move towards a new theme.

But sisterly reason (symbolised by Minerva and related

goddesses in the Celtic-Classical mythologies) cannot prevail, and the personal or sexual love of Guendoloena is called upon to restrain Merlin in his flight from reason back to wild fervour. 'But he spurned her prayers and would not stay, nor would he, as he was accustomed to do, look upon her with a joyful face.' The interplay between wife and sister is again suggested here; it is as if Merlin has foreseen his wife's acceptance of another man.

It must be stressed strongly that there is not a psychological implication of incest in our magical or transpersonal interpretation; the wife or lover and the sister, as said earlier, are aspects of a female divinity in their most primal form. In the *Vita* we have a complex interweaving of these aspects, shown by the personalities of Ganieda and Gwendoloena. In other Celtic tales that involve Merlin or his Scottish counterpart Lailoken, the roles of lover and sister are interchanged without altering the major themes of madness, personal love, and impersonal or transpersonal consciousness.

Guendoleona is willing to accompany Merlin to the woods, but he rejects her company strongly. Sexual love cannot conjoin with the prophetic madness at this stage. The situation is constantly supervised by queen Ganieda, Merlin's sister. While Guendoloena tears her hair and rolls upon the ground in fruitless ritual despair, it is Ganieda who asks the key question: 'What shall she do . . . shall she marry again or do you bid her remain a widow, or go with you wherever you are going?'

The sequence of Guendoloena's choices is revealing; once Merlin has left for the prophetic life, she is a widow. Traditionally initiates into the Mysteries are regarded as dead, they have died to the world and become reborn to a new world. In primitive rituals worldwide the symbolic death is often accompanied by a form of ritual sacrifice and endurance, a direct expression of the metaphysical properties symbolised by the Threefold Death.[1]

The choices that remain to Merlin's wife are expressed by his sister, and once again we have the interplay between two women who seem to symbolise aspects of both consciousness and of the divine; one is reason and instruction, while the other is passion. Yet, as in the drama of Rhydderch's court, they may interchange their roles if they wish to do so. From this point on, however, Guendoloena becomes a stereotype, and she is soon to disappear from the tale altogether. Merlin begins slowly and painfully to replace personal love with a more subtle transpersonal pursuit of wisdom.

Merlin rejects his wife with a curious speech, in which astrological overtones seem to provide a rationale for his rejection. 'I do not want a cow that pours out water in a broad fountain like the Urn of the Virgin in flood.' This is either a high-flown simile for his wife's excessive tears, or it refers to a stellar theme which has not survived Geoffrey's translation or retelling. In *The Prophecies* the Virgin is described leaping shamelessly upon the Centaur (Sagittarius) and losing her virtue;[2] there may be some interplay between this cosmic image and that woodland image of Merlin appearing upon a stag's back and leading goats to his wife's marriage with another man, an image which we shall examine shortly.

Merlin finally gives his wife permission to remarry, but with the reservation that he may take revenge upon the new husband, and with the promise that he will furnish gifts at the wedding in person.[3] This threatening promise bodes ill for any lover of Guendoloena, and we are ready for a classic revenge theme. The resolution, however, comes in completely magical terms, in which Merlin's threat is carried out in a most graphic and unusual manner.

MERLIN'S FIRST SIGN OF STAR-LORE

So Merlin returns to the woods, forsaking his worldly rulership; Guendoloena remarries according to Merlin's permission.

In the verses which follow, we have the introduction of a simple star-watching and astrological element, overtly stated for the first time. This marks the turning point of a progression that has slowly crept upon us in the early stages of the biography; Merlin is now advanced far enough upon his prophetic path to make direct utterances and observations, something which he could not do before due to the consuming passion of his first frenzy after the dreadful battle, and his violent return to a primal life.

In this scene his intellectual capacity is beginning to merge with his seership, and he is able to interpret stellar or planetary signs consciously. Prior to this stage, which arises after the ritual drama of the Threefold Death incident, he could only bewail the passage of the seasons; now he can read that passage upon the mirror of the night sky, and rise above his discomfort and confusion.

Once again, Merlin has reached the hilltop; the resulting images are not borrowed from his *Prophecies*, a borrowing which develops in a later section, but are readings of his own present which he uses to see afar. This is a development of the simple far-seeing in the leaf-love incident,[4] for the imagery is now linked to stellar events. In other words, he is seeing through space and not through time at this stage of his development as a seer. Just as he sees through space first and then through time in respect of the Threefold Death incident, now he sees through space in a more complex manner, just as sections of *The Prophecies* are reiterated to show a more developed seeing-through-time in a later section of the *Vita*[5]

Venus shining with a double ray becomes a symbol of his wife remarrying, and this is harmonically related to changes of the ruler on the throne. Mars and Venus are paired together in traditional astrology as in mythology: the god of war and the goddess of love.

The balanced far-seeing is not a mere contrivance, for we find similar harmonic links running through *The Prophecies* in which historic events and persons are sometimes inseparable from magical or even spiritual symbols; the outer and inner factors and energies are the mutual opposites of one another, yet are inseparably linked. We might approach this in another way, and suggest that just as Mars shows a change of the ruling king of Britain, so does the feminine planet of Venus show a change of the ruling direction of Merlin's personal love,

Guendoloena. Merlin then determines to deliver his promised gift.

MERLIN AS LORD OF THE ANIMALS

Merlin's gift to his ex-wife is not a simple one, and once again we find him in the role of a wild power of nature. He assembles a herd of stags, deer and she-goats, and seated upon a stag himself, presents these as his gift.

There is a close link here to imagery found in the *Mabinogion* ('The Lady of The Fountain') where a giant black man herds and controls stags, is the possessor of awesome power, and defends a sacred spring.[6] Merlin has the attributes of control over stags and the relationship to a magical spring, established already in the narrative but developed later during the scene in which he is finally cured of madness.[7] We also find an implication of superhuman strength in this stag scene, for he tears the horns from his mount and hurls them with such force that his rival is killed instantly, even though he was watching 'from a lofty window'.

No further mention is made of the bridegroom, or of Merlin's wife, after this curious dramatic scene. They have been wiped out of the narrative, which moves on to develop mystical themes.

The new husband is, in fact, a mere cypher; he cannot replace the primal power represented by Merlin who destroys him when they come into contact. From this point on, in the magical sense of the story, an unpolarised and incomplete flower maiden (Guendoloena) simply vanishes like the blossoms from which her counterpart was made by another Welsh magician, Math the son of Mathonwy.[8]

The theme is again related to polarity and partnerships: in this dream-like journey of Merlin from madness to spiritual clarity, he outgrows certain aspects of his psyche, and they vanish or are destroyed. The seemingly callous nature of this adventure is due to the symbolic language; the psychic or magical units are shown through personal characterisation in the hallowed traditional manner. In this way they act directly upon the consciousness without intellectual interface; we all know intuitively what the stag-scene means, even if our level of understanding differs or we cannot explain it in intellectual terms.

As mentioned above, the horns were not only a symbol of nature power, connected to the Lord of the Animals and the Wild Hunt; they were also a symbol of the man deceived or sexually betrayed by his wife. Here the generative element of the symbols comes to the fore, with the horns playing a phallic role. But this is only the first and most obvious level of the meaning; it is not the only level, nor is it the most important one. The wearing of horns was found in traditional ceremonies across Europe, and the entire complex of images in which Merlin directs stags, tears the horns from a stag, uses horns as a weapon against a rival lover is very similar to elements found in mummers plays and ritual dance dramas.

As early as the fourth century AD Saint Augustine sternly opposed 'that most filthy habit of dressing up as a horse or stag'; in the twentieth century the people of Cornwall still do so, and still sing 'Take no scorn to wear the horns, they were a sign ere you were born/Your father's father wore them, and your father wore them too'. In this case the animal symbolism refers to death, resurrection and fertility rituals enacted at the opening of May, the ancient festival of the Pleiades (Beltane) and the originally pagan image of St George, a wild green man in the sacred woods.[9]

To Geoffrey's audience there would be both a sexual double meaning, possibly a joke, and a clear link to traditional rites and half-forgotten pagan symbols still kept alive in song, drama, and tales.

Merlin's rapid flight on the back of his stag leads him to fall into the river where servants capture him, bind him and carry him back to his sister, who once again appears as a controlling element to whom Merlin is joined willing or not. The fishing of a seer from a river has certain parallels with tales in which a holy and prophetic child is fished out of the water, and taken to the court of the king.[10]

Figure 6 shows the relationships between various characters, set upon the Wheel of Life and the Four Seasons.

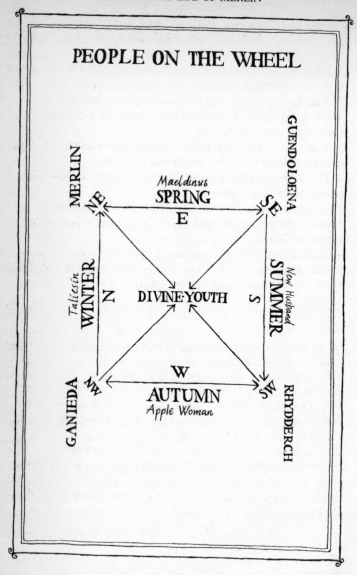

Figure 6 *People on the Wheel*

PEOPLE ON THE WHEEL

1 Merlin-Guendoloena: lovers; winter-spring; NE-SE; sexual polar relationship.
2 Merlin-Rhydderch: equalising opposites; hermit and wildman/king and man of the world; NE-SW; qualities balance in centre of Wheel.
3 Ganieda-Merlin: sister-brother; autumn-winter; NW-NE; non-sexual but polarised relationship.
4 Ganieda-Rhydderch: lovers; autumn-summer; NW-SW; sexual polar relationship.
5 Ganieda-Guendoloena: equalising opposites; Flower Female and Wisdom Female; NW-SE; qualities balance in centre of Wheel.
6 Guendoloena-Rhydderch; no relationship stated, but similar to that of brother and sister (spring-summer; SE-SW; non-sexual but polarised relationship).

The qualities of each character are outlined in Appendix II: *People*.

To the power or energy pattern shown above, we could add the following people:

1 Taliesin: north, instructor of wisdom. Mediator between Minerva, goddess of wisdom, and Merlin, the candidate for initiation. Minerva is the archetype or goddess-form behind Ganieda. (Element of earth.)
2 Maeldinus: east, wild man of the woods, power of prophetic madness, rising forces of nature. Symbol of fervent spirit. (Element of air.)
3 Youth: centre, victim of Threefold Death. Fusion of all characters.

Taliesin reflects wisdom north-south, while Maeldinus transmits energy east-west.

If the pattern is read sunwise (ESWN) each character merges into the other, sharing harmonic attributes but changing outer gender (Guendoloena, Rhydderch, Ganieda, Merlin).

If the pattern is read across the poles (as in Figure 6) various interactions arise which are narrated within the *Vita*.

The shadowy figures of the *Apple Woman* (west) and the *New Husband* (south) may be added to complete the pattern. The Apple Woman is a mysterious power figure who offers magical fruit, while the New Husband is a male stereotype sought by Guendoloena. Each of these figures are likely to be faint resonances of pagan deities: The Goddess of Life and the God of Procreation. (Elements of water and fire.)

CHAPTER 7
Merlin's second return

No offices of Janus shall return hereafter, but the gate being shut shall remain hidden in the crannies of Ariadne.
The Prophecies of Merlin.

My threshold is constructed out of every feeling of fear to which you are still accessible, out of every shrinking from the power which will take over to itself the complete responsibility for all your deeds and thoughts. So long as you have still any fear of that self-government of your fate, all that belongs to this threshold has not yet been built into it . . . seek not, then, to pass my threshold until you feel yourself liberated from all fear, ready for the highest responsibility.
The Guardian proclaims his significance: Rudolph Steiner.

While fleeing from the scene of the death of Guendoloena's new husband, Merlin falls from the back of his stag into the river, where the servants of Ganieda catch him and carry him back to court.

Once again Rhydderch tries to distract Merlin, by taking him to view the market-place. The prophet laughs twice, once when looking at a door-keeper who begs for alms, and again at a young man buying new shoes and leather patches. He exchanges his freedom for the reasons behind his laughter, and reveals the secrets of both individuals through his far-sight.

MERLIN'S SECOND RETURN

The prophet, captured in this way, became sad and wanted to go back to the woods, and he fought to break his bonds

89

and refused to smile or to take food or drink, and by his sadness he made his sister sad. Rhydderch, therefore, seeing him drive all joy from him and refuse to taste of the banquets that had been prepared for him, took pity on him and ordered him to be led out into the city, through the market-place among the people, in the hope that he might be cheered up by going and seeing the novelties that were being sold there.

After he had been taken out and was going away from the palace he saw before a door a servant of a poor appearance, the door-keeper, asking with trembling lips of all the passers-by some money with which to get his clothes mended. The prophet thereupon stood still and laughed, wondering at the poor man. When he had gone on from here he saw a young man holding some new shoes and buying some pieces of leather to patch them with. Then he laughed again and refused to go further through the market-place to be stared at by the people he was watching. But he yearned for the woods, toward which he frequently looked back, and to which, although forbidden, he tried to direct his steps.

The servants returned home and told that he had laughed twice and also that he had tried to get away to the woods. Rhydderch, who wished to know what he had meant by his laughter, quickly gave orders for his bonds to be loosed and gave him permission to go back to his accustomed woods if only he would explain why he laughed. The prophet, now quite joyful, answered, 'The door-keeper was sitting outside the doors in well-worn clothing and kept asking those who went by to give him something to buy clothes with, just as though he had been a pauper, and all the time he was secretly a rich man and had under him hidden piles of coins. That is what I laughed at; turn up the ground under him and you will find coins preserved there for a long time. From there they led me further toward the market-place and I saw a man buying some shoes and also some patches so that after the shoes were worn out and had holes in them from use he might mend them and make them fit for service again. This too I laughed at since the poor man will not be able to use the shoes nor,' he added, 'the patches, since he is already drowned in the waves and is floating toward the shore; go and you will see.' Rhydderch, wishing to test the man's sayings, ordered his servants to go quickly along the bank of the river, so that if they should chance to find such a man drowned by the shore they might at once bring him word. They obeyed the king's orders, for going along the river they found a drowned man in a waste patch of sand, and returned home and reported the fact to him. But the king meanwhile, after sending away the door-keeper, had dug and turned up the ground and found a treasure placed under it, and laughingly he worshipped the prophet.

MERLIN'S SECOND RETURN

Merlin is bound by the servants, and taken back to his sister. Once again he refuses to be cheerful, and King Rhydderch seeks, as before, to divert him and draw him back into the regular world.

The narrative now draws upon a tale which has some clearly oriental equivalents; Merlin laughs at apparently ordinary incidents while he is being taken around the market-place. In each case, that of a door-keeper begging and of a young man buying new shoes and patches, the prophet exhibits his heightened powers of perception. Similar tales are found in Jewish folklore, Arabic entertainments or wisdom tales, and in the Talmud. How the material reached Geoffrey, or in what form, is a matter of speculation; by the twelfth century there was certainly an exchange of lore between Europe and the East, probably on a greater scale than we commonly assume and possibly separate from best known sources such as returning Crusaders.[1]

In *The Prophecies* there is an absence of Arabic astronomy or astrology; the star-lore is mainly native British or Greek. This absence is likely to be due to the oral traditional source on which Geoffrey drew, a source predating *The History* in which *The Prophecies* are included, probably by several centuries. By the time Geoffrey wrote the *Vita*, however, drawing upon similar oral bardic sources, he had also 'collected' tales from an Eastern source and these are included to represent Merlin's growing powers.

The alternative possibility, which demands serious consideration and cuts across the matter of literary derivation, is that such tales arise spontaneously in the human consciousness. Connections between wisdom tales may not be entirely a matter of literary or cultural transmission, but of the dream-flow in which such tales are crystallised out of common *environmental, psychic,* and *spiritual* experiences.

The first level, that of the environment or land, will colour the basic modes of expression of any theme most distinctively, while the second begins to form relationships with similar motifs in a cross-cultural manner due to inherent relationships between the human psyche regardless of its physical or cultural location. At this second stage the differences are still very considerable. By the third stage, spiritual or transcendental, we find that themes fuse together to state a mode or quality of experience which is known worldwide, albeit expressed through the filters of the preceding levels. There are no hard and fast boundaries between these theoretical levels of consciousness, and often they cut across one another (see Figure 7).

In a narrative poem drawn mainly from British and classical traditions, with the major portion of the material being Celtic, Geoffrey's insertion of an Eastern tale is all the more remarkable.

In our context of the narrative as a description and practical guide to inner growth, symbolised by the figure of Merlin, the two images (the beggar who sits on a hoard of gold, and the youth who buys new shoes and patches for the shoes shortly before drowning) are classic wisdom tales. They not only act as examples of Merlin's own foresight (the shoes) and heightened perceptions (the hoard), but are wisdom motifs in their own right. Each image demonstrates an aspect of our human condition: the beggar who unwittingly sits upon great riches, and the youth who plans a long life yet dies immediately.

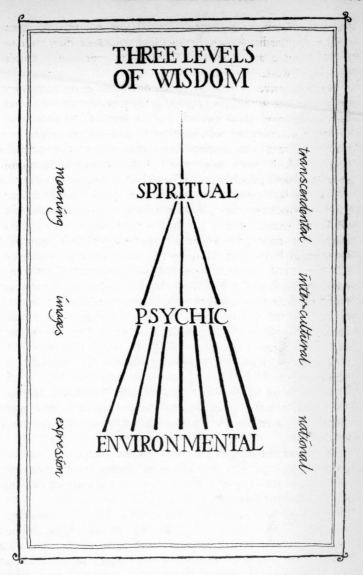

Figure 7 *Three levels of wisdom*

Such tales form an important part of educational and mystical lore disseminated by word of mouth, and there are further symbolic levels to each of these apparently trivial items which are worth exploring briefly.

The Impoverished Door-keeper is a clear symbol of the human consciousness, particularly of the personality (in the modern sense). He begs money from passers-by 'to mend his clothes'; we might say that he seeks to feed his self-image by drawing approval from others. The significance of door-keeper is not trivial; he is firstly a symbol of the personality that sits upon the threshold of a greater and richer consciousness, the hidden hoard of gold, while convinced of its own weakness or poverty and constantly seeking outward support instead of looking within or below for hidden wealth.

In medieval culture door-keeping still held the ancient sanctity with which it was endowed in earlier times. A door-keeper or porter was both the lowest and highest office, for he admitted people to the hall or castle. This role is still found in ritual situations such as ceremonial magic or Masonic lodges today. Ultimately it derives from the potent image of the *Guardian*, clearly described in its divine aspect by Merlin in *The Prophecies*.[2]

The deluded personality is that fragment of the door-keeper furthest removed from this cosmic archetypical power of guardianship or opening/closing, yet still sits upon untold wealth and power. In this allegorical sense we could add that when the king 'sends the door-keeper away' and digs up the gold, he is asserting our royal right of consciousness to be self-controlling, and not merely at the whim of the beggar element of the personality. Thereafter he laughingly worships Merlin, who represents the deep prophetic or intuitive powers that lead us towards inner freedom.

The Youth with new shoes represents the folly of attempting to secure a 'future'. He buys shoes *and* patches for the shoes, assuming that he will ensure a safe and comfortable ride for himself under conditions which do not change radically. He is following the usual pattern of human behaviour in which we act as if our wishful projections of life are in fact life itself.

While the first image, of the door-keeper, concerns levels of consciousness, the second is of the transitory nature of life and aspirations. The youth is found drowned 'in a waste patch of sand' by the seashore; his spirit set out upon the ocean of eternity, leaving his absurd image of himself behind.

The moral and religious aspect of each of these exemplary tales would have been very strong indeed to Geoffrey's medieval audience, though we tend to sneer at such symbolism today. Not only do the tales act in the *Vita* as proof of Merlin's powers of perception, but they also show him to be a purveyor of *wisdom* over and above *information*. The short scene of attempted distraction in the market-place has become transformed into a lesson in spiritual values. The servants and king have attempted to trivialise Merlin's madness by merely entertaining him or keeping him occupied, and he has leapt beyond the serial activities bound by time to find situations and personal examples that stand this materialist attitude upon its head.

Once again, Merlin returns to society, hates and rejects what he finds there, and leaves for the wildwood. After his second return, however, he now enters upon a co-operative venture with his sister; mere running wild in the woods has been transformed into an ordered prophetic consciousness by his experiences.

CHAPTER 8
Merlin's Observatory

The Twelve Houses of the Stars shall lament the irregular
excursions of their inmates.

The Prophecies of Merlin.

Ganieda seeks to restrain Merlin from returning to the woods,
and he agrees that his mode of life should change. He requests
her to build an Observatory, with a house for winter shelter,
where he can watch the stars and have detailed notes taken by
scribes. He spends the Summer close to nature, but the Winter
in the Observatory.

MERLIN'S OBSERVATORY

After these things had happened the prophet was making
haste to go to the woods he was accustomed to, hating the
people in the city. The queen advised him to stay with her
and to put off his desired trip to the woods until the cold of
white winter, which was then at hand, should be over, and
summer should return again with its tender fruits on which
he could live while the weather grew warm from the sun. He
refused, and desirous of departing and scorning the winter he
said to her, 'O dear sister, why do you labor to hold me
back? Winter with his tempests cannot frighten me, nor icy
Boreas when he rages with his cruel blasts and suddenly
injures the flocks of sheep with hail; neither does Auster
disturb me when its rain clouds shed their waters. Why
should I not seek the deserted groves and the green
woodlands? Content with a little I can endure the frost.
There under the leaves of the trees among the odorous

blossoms I shall take pleasure in lying through the summer; but lest I lack food in winter you might build me a house in the woods and have servants in it to wait on me and prepare me food when the ground refuses to produce grain or the trees fruit. Before the other buildings build me a remote one with seventy doors and as many windows through which I may watch fire-breathing Phoebus and Venus and the stars gliding from the heavens by night, all of whom shall show me what is going to happen to the people of the kingdom. And let the same number of scribes be at hand, trained to take my dictation, and let them be attentive to record my prophecy on their tablets. You too are to come often, dear sister, and then you can relieve my hunger with food and drink.' After he had finished speaking he departed hastily for the woods.

His sister obeyed him and built the place he had asked for, and the other houses and whatever else he had bid her. But he, while the apples remained and Phoebus was ascending higher through the stars, rejoiced to remain beneath the leaves and to wander through the groves with their soothing breezes. Then winter came, harsh with icy winds, and despoiled the ground and the trees of all their fruit, and Merlin lacked food because the rains were at hand, and he came, sad and hungry, to the aforesaid place. Thither the queen often came and rejoiced to bring her brother both food and drink. He, after he had refreshed himself with various kinds of edibles, would arise and express his approval of his sister. Then wandering about the house he would look at the stars while he prophesied things like these which he knew were going to come to pass.

MERLIN'S OBSERVATORY

The building of a complex dedicated to star-watching marks a full revolution of Merlin's spiralling journey. He is again at Winter, and Ganieda attempts to restrain his flight into the ascetic life of the woodland hermit. A working arrangement is made betwen Merlin and his sister, the prophetic consciousness and the educational or enabling consciousness.

Although this complex of buildings has obvious suggestions of the monastic settlement, it is not religious in a Christian sense; it is devoted to watching the stars for purposes of prophecy. Merlin has a remote or separated building with seventy doors and seventy windows, set apart from the dwelling-house and servants' quarters; it is Ganieda who supervises both the building and the operation of this complex. A body of scribes, also seventy, take notes from Merlin's observation of the stars which show him 'what is going to happen to the people of the kingdom'.[1]

There are various ways in which we can interpret this scene; primarily it gives substance to an established tradition that Merlin gained many of his prophetic insights from star-lore. His stellar wisdom is not identical to modern astrology, and is defined more fully in The Prophecies. But such a precise description of Merlin's observatory may come from an established source within the general flow of common traditions such as those found in The History; when such traditional images are read correctly they are found to link harmonically with historical (factual) matters.

The famous incident of Merlin and Stonehenge is an excellent example, in which the prophet brought the stones from Ireland as a great memorial burial site. Although the hard facts may be false, this tale in the History[2] represents a tradition in which Stonehenge comes from a land to the far West, is associated with death and the Otherworld, and is linked to the magical practices of pre-Christian cultures through the figure of Merlin. Taken in such a light, Geoffrey's account fits very well with the modern account made by archaeology; the stones come in part from Wales, burials are associated with such sites generally, and their origination is likely to be magical/religious.

A further element, now well attested though still debated, is that stone circles are aligned to the rising or setting of certain stars and planets. As with the Stonehenge image connected to Merlin as a magician and stellar seer, so with the Observatory image. It represents a tradition deriving from beliefs connected to pagan and ancient cultures, in which structures were built or employed to symbolise stellar wisdom, to make observations, and to make calculations.[3]

In a dream-like manner, tradition has preserved the echoes of a culture or cultures far removed in time from the medieval period; echoes which have been at least partially proven by the work of modern archaeologists and scientists. In short, the ancients built special sites to observe the stars, and this practice was symbolised by Merlin as late as the twelfth century.

A similar image occurs in *The History* in Geoffrey's description of the Court of Arthur at Caerleon, though the link to prophecy is less obvious.[4] In terms of an oral Celtic tradition, such as those from which the *Vita* and *The History* were substantially drawn, the Observatory represents at least two strata of cultural history. The first is that ancient dream-enfolded memory of the purpose of the standing stones and circles; stones which would have been the subject of wide-spread superstition and legend in the medieval period, as we find from Geoffrey's account of Stonehenge. The second would be much closer in a cultural historical sense, for it preserves the educational and prophetic function of the bard, which derives in turn from the pagan Druids, who persisted in Wales until at least the first century AD.

A related tradition is preserved by Geoffrey in his retelling of the story of King Bladud, who appears in both *The History* and the *Vita*, who flew through the air, practiced necromancy, and founded not only the Temple of Minerva at Aquae Sulis (Bath) but also a college or teaching establishment.[5] Such traditions have preserved the function of the Druidic or Celtic king and priest, albeit in a confused manner. But the confusion arises only in the pedantically factual logical mind that demands literal evidence; traditional evidence is symbolic, dreamlike, and intimately attuned to crisp visual images. The myth of Bladud, for example, is amply confirmed by modern archaeology, although the site of the Temple of the Minerva had been buried for several centuries in Geoffrey's day.

Merlin's Observatory is all the more remarkable for the

purity of its directly pagan purpose; orthodox religion is not involved in any way whatsoever. It sets the scene not only for the series of prophecies which follow (mainly but not entirely drawn from the early book of *The Prophecies* included in *The History*), but for the educational or initiatory teaching of Taliesin in a later scene, under the instruction of Minerva. As we have suggested, Ganieda is an expression or personal representation of a goddess image similar to Minerva; this is why she builds and supervises the Observatory. Her role is not that of a domestic sister tending to her mad brother, but of an enabling power.

Numerical symbolism of the Observatory

It is possible that the number seventy is not merely a poetic conceit, and interacts with the traditional function of ancient sites and their (now proven) mathematical orientation to certain stars and planets. In this context we should first remember that such observatories are not merely the remnants of a Celtic tradition linked to Druidic lore or prehistoric structures; they are also found in developed cultures of other lands. The best-known example of course are those of ancient Egypt, and of South America, where remarkable structures were built to express theories about the relationship between the stars, planets, and the mysterious Otherworld. Merlin's Observatory is not merely a derivative image from tradition or literary sources, it represents a pattern of consciousness and of cultural expression known in many forms from the most simple to the most sophisticated, and found worldwide throughout every age or civilisation. In this sense alone it is of prime importance in the *Vita* as a manifestation of the development of human awareness. Humankind looks not only within, but to the universe at large for harmonious insights into the meaning of existence.[6]

The number seventy may be derived from the basic symbolism of the Seven Planets. Planetary attributes are repeatedly referred to in both *The Prophecies* and the *Vita*, and the Elemental/Planetary system was an accepted and basic worldview in the medieval period, deriving from a fusion of classical and western European cultural inheritance. Arabic astrology began to permeate the west during Geoffrey's lifetime or perhaps slightly earlier, revitalising knowledge which had remained relatively static during the Dark Ages.

The basic planetary attributes have remained constant for many thousands of years, and are employed today as psychological symbols rather than energies that influence mankind upon the planet Earth.

The Observatory introduces us to this type of theory, leads into the section of pseudo-historical prophecies, but also prepares us for the more detailed Elemental exposition which follows, acting as Merlin's final instruction in the Mysteries prior to his cure at a magical spring.

Not only do we have the traditional Seven Planets, but a harmonic link between these planets and the seven power centres or psychic centres of the human entity. The perception through sevenfold doors and windows may be an image of such a system within the individual seer.

In astrology, each sign of the Zodiac is divided in three Decanates, each of ten degrees. If we find Merlin viewing each of the planets in turn through a door or window representing a degree, we have the figure of 7×10. One scribe attends each degree of observation for each planet in each Decanate. The Decanates were used historically by both the Egyptians and the Greeks to locate fixed stars, which system may have been part of the loose assemblage of ancient astrology found in *The Prophecies*, where Greek symbolism plays a strong role.

The Observatory, with its seventy windows, seventy doors, and seventy scribes is theoretically a very precise and minute apparatus for accurate observation of the night skies, relating directly to actual astronomical practices in the ancient world, and symbolically to the Elemental and Planetary system of metaphysics which acted as the philosophical and psychological foundation of Western culture. This same system has world-wide currency in an attenuated form even today, and formed the basis of several major civilisations in both the East and the

West. The Observatory is a property of consciousness seeking to create order and predictive order upon the cosmos. It is the materialisation of the cycles shown by Merlin's own adventure and his prophecies (both in the *Vita* and the earlier book of *Prophecies*; it is a microcosmic model of the macrocosmic order.[7]

Finally we should remember that the *Vita* and *The Prophecies* both derive from wisdom teachings which are essentially British or Celtic; the expression of a goddess as Minerva (the *Vita*) or Ariadne (*The Prophecies*) is due to Geoffrey's classical writing for a partially educated audience, and in keeping with the precedents of style demanded of a medieval churchman. To both the mythology and the astronomy/astrology we must apply flexible rules of derivation; the evidence of native tradition is at least as strong as the literary derivation from Greek or Roman classical and post-classical sources.[8]

CHAPTER 9

I *Merlin's prophetic history*
II *Lament for King Rhydderch*

> Merlin, by delivering these and many other prophecies,
> caused in all that were present an admiration at the double
> meaning of his utterances. But Vortigern above all others
> both admired and applauded the wisdom and prophetical
> spirit. . . . That age had produced none that ever talked in
> such a manner.
>
> *The History of The British Kings.*

From his astrological observations and prophetic power,
Merlin utters a long sequence of British history. This concludes
with knowledge of the death of King Rhydderch, and of the
arrival of the bard Taliesin from a learned school in Brittany.
Ganieda leaves the Observatory and returns to the court, to
mourn and lament for her husband the dead king.

MERLIN'S PROPHETIC HISTORY

The scene of the Observatory, and the employment of both
stellar observation and mundane astrology prepare the reader
or listener for this directly predictive scene, in which a semi-
historical summary is given by Merlin of his Prophecies uttered
to King Vortigern, 'explaining to him the mystic war of the two
dragons when we sat on the banks of the drained pool'. This
sequence is drawn from *The History*, where *The Prophecies*
take up two chapters, and form a concentrated separate entity
within the main text.[1]
There are a number of differences or expansions in this

sequence of the *Vita*, which have been commented upon by scholars.[2] One significant point which has been passed over in literary commentary, however, is that the *Vita* prophecies are entirely 'historic'; they do not contain any of the mystical vision or apocalyptic symbolism found in the larger text incorporated into Geoffrey's early work, *The History*. In this later reworking, Geoffrey has concentrated entirely upon the historical (to us pseudo-historical) progression which supports the time-scale of events as traditionally set out by historians of his own period; *The Prophecies* have been quite tightly edited.

In our examination of *The Prophecies*, mystical and pseudo-historical events or symbols were found to be intermixed.[3] Sometimes the mixture was random, while in other sections there were coherent but recondite themes displayed. Mixtures of this sort are typical of verses or teachings drawn from tradition, in which the tradition is of sufficient power and authority to remain revered and unedited, even after it may have become confused or corrupt. The most obvious parallel is that of the Old Testament, where many quite obscure and irrelevant motifs, ritual observations, assertions of dogma and the like are preserved from Hebrew tradition because of the inherent sanctity of the overall book. Much of this lore was confused even before it became Westernised, and the Talmud is still the subject of debate and commentary today just as it was in the living traditions of previous centuries.

By the time Geoffrey assembled the *Vita*, he was recounting a series of poems or tales relating to Merlin as a figure who demonstrated the Celtic magical or proto-psychological wisdom: stories which were known in both Scotland and Wales, though in varying forms. The mystical symbolism is no longer offered in the form of a hallowed traditional sequence as in *The Prophecies*, but in the expanded example of Merlin's own inner growth and final salvation from madness.

The prophecies offered here, therefore, are really a type of required 'padding' or corroboration much beloved by medieval writers and story-tellers. Geoffrey has removed the obscure elements and retained the historical ones for reasons of neatness, but also to act as a balance to the mystical lore expressed throughout the *Vita*. This is straight prediction and far-seeing, nothing more. It leads us directly to the death of King Rhydderch, and the invitation to Taliesin who has returned from Brittany.[4] These two themes bring us back to the narrative flow of the biography.

LAMENT FOR KING RHYDDERCH

Ganieda returned home and found that Taliesin had returned and the prince was dead and the servants were sad. She fell down lamenting among her friends and tore her hair and cried, 'Women, lament with me the death of Rhydderch and weep for a man such as our earth has not produced hitherto in our age so far as we know. He was a lover of peace, for he so ruled a fierce people that no violence was done to any one by any one else. He treated the holy priest with just moderation and permitted the highest and the lowest to be governed by law. He was generous, for he gave away much and kept scarcely anything. He was all things to all men, doing whatever was seemly; flower of knights, glory of kings, pillar of the kingdom. Who is me! for what you were – now so unexpectedly you have become food for worms, and your body moulders in the urn. Is this the bed prepared for you after fine silks? Is it true that your white flesh and royal limbs will be covered by a cold stone, that you will be nothing but dust and bones? So it is, for the miserable lot of mankind goes on throughout the years so that they cannot be brought back to their former estate. Therefore there is no profit in the bravery of the transient world that flees and returns, deceives and injures the mighty. The bee anoints with its honey what it afterwards stings. So also those whom the glory of the world caresses as it departs it deceives and smites with its disagreeable sting. That which excels is of brief duration, what it has does not endure; like running water everything that is of service passes away. What is a rose if it blushes, a snowy lily if it blooms, a man or a horse or anything else if it is fair! These things should be referred to the Creator, not to the world. Happy therefore are those who remain firm in a pious heart and serve God and renounce the world. To them Christ who reigns without end, the Creator of all things, shall grant to enjoy perpetual honor. Therefore I leave you, ye nobles, ye lofty walls, household gods, sweet sons, and all the things of the world. In company with my brother I shall dwell in the woods and shall worship God with a joyful heart, clothed in a black mantle.' So she spoke, giving her husband his due, and she inscribed on his tomb this verse, 'Rhydderch the Generous, than whom there was no one more generous in the world, a great man rests in this small urn.'

LAMENT FOR KING RHYDDERCH

Merlin's predictions have flowed into the present of the narrative, and it is now Ganieda who, seemingly for the first time, experiences the suffering of loss. Her earlier lack of fidelity to her husband is completely forgotten (and irrelevant) for it was of the order of ritual drama not personal history. The Lament that she utters for her dead husband is a beautiful poem which transcends her personal loss, and introduces a number of customary and traditional reflections upon the brevity of human life. The tone is similar to that of the messenger's poem uttered to Merlin earlier, and the symbolism is shared in some lines. It is the death of Rhydderch which prompts Ganieda to retire to the woods and join with her brother in the mystic life.

This poem is significant in another way, for it is Ganieda who refers to 'Christ who reigns without end, the Creator of all things . . .' A formally religious note is brought in for the first time, but this is no mere sop to orthodoxy, nor does it in any way change the developing pagan classical philosophy of the narrative; indeed, Ganieda immediately bids farewell not only to her noble chiefs and sweet children, but also to her household gods. This mixture reflects very accurately the innocent or persistent presence of paganism amidst orthodoxy;

it may be a confusion of symbolism from Geoffrey's traditional oral source, or it may actually reflect a typical Celtic practice. Curious images are found even today in Ireland and Brittany, called saints, but clearly older gods and goddesses.

We may interpret this poem on two levels, that of Ganieda as queen and her renunciation of the material life for the spiritual or prophetic life, and that of Rhydderch as a symbol for the material kingship or values of the material world, a role which he has repeatedly enacted in his dealings with Merlin. Both levels are interrelated through the person of Ganieda.

Rhydderch's good qualities listed in the Lament are the classic requirements of a good king; these qualities recur again and again in literature from the medieval period onwards. But he also played the part of captor and tempter to Merlin, not in any covertly evil sense, but as a king who represented the balanced worldly values in which prophetic fervour plays no part . . . until proven accurate!

Rhydderch also acts as a stereotypical male in the scene leading up to the Threefold Death; Ganieda is not tied to Rhydderch in the way that Guendoloena the sexual female must be tied to a male to be complete. It is Rhydderch's death, in fact, that fulfils his role as king, and we may be hearing a faint resonance from an earlier culture in which kingship was sacred and sacrificial, reflecting the power of a god who died and was reborn.

The Lament is divided into two parts, personal memorial, and impersonal philosophy or mystical reflection. The turning or spiralling theme which is clearly epitomised by Merlin, his mad rush through the seasons and his early laments for the presence of winter, is reiterated here: 'so the world's glory turns again and deceives those it has caressed, piercing hard with its unwelcome sting.'

The reflections upon the transience of lilies and roses reminds us of the floral nature of Guendoloena, who has been passed over for a different and mystical life. The message is not hard to find: either the individual soul must outgrow the transient cycles of nature, or the cycles of nature will carry the individual to death. Guendoloena, the flower woman, was considered a

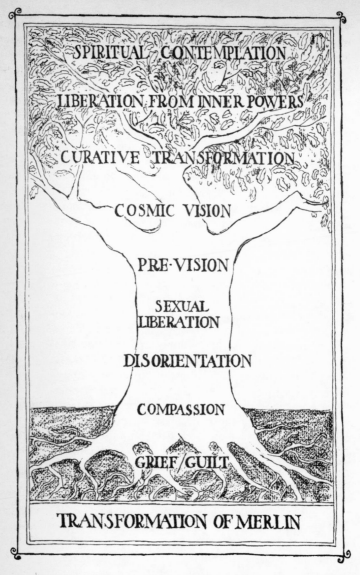

Figure 8 *The transformation of Merlin*

widow when Merlin withdrew to the woods; to live in the inner or mystical life is to die to the outer or material life (see Figure 8).

The Lament concludes with Ganieda donning her black cloak and joining her brother in the woods.

CHAPTER 10
The Creation of the World

The Four Winds shall fight together with a dreadful blast and their sound shall reach to the stars.
The Prophecies of Merlin.

Discover thou what it is, the strong creature from before the flood/Without flesh without bone without vein without blood . . . It frequently comes proceeding from the heat of the Sun and the coldness of the Moon/ . . . One being has prepared it out of all creatures, by a tremendous blast.
Taliesin's Riddle of the Wind.

Taliesin, newly returned from the school of wisdom in Brittany, comes to visit Merlin. Merlin repeats his most important question, apparently asking 'What is weather?' The answer is a description of the Creation of the World, not just the planet Earth but the entire cosmos, both the greater World of the stars and the lesser World of our planet. Both are shown to be harmonically related.

After revealing the links between the stars and the seas and lands, Taliesin then proceeds to the mysteries of the Other-world, which is a magical realm within the Earth, or across a sea, that leads into another dimension. The legend of King Arthur resting in the Fortunate Isle, waiting to return, is the culmination of the vision. Certain strange characters of mythical origin are introduced, and their powers are hinted at or openly described.

CREATION OF THE WORLD

Elements and circles

Meanwhile Taliesin had come to see Merlin the prophet who had sent for him to find out what caused wind or rainstorms, for both together were drawing near and the clouds were thickening. He drew the following illustrations under the guidance of Minerva his associate.

'Out of nothing the Creator of the world produced *four elements* that they might be the prior cause as well as the material for creating all things when they were joined together in harmony: the *heaven* which He adorned with *stars* and which stands on high and embraces everything like the shells surrounding a nut; then He made the *air*, fit for forming sounds, through the medium of which day and night present the stars; the *sea* which girds the land in four circles, and with its mighty refluence so strikes the air as to generate the *winds* which are said to be four in number; as a foundation He placed the earth, standing by its own strength and not lightly moved, which is divided into five parts, whereof the middle one is not habitable because of the heat and the two furthest are shunned because of their cold. To the last two He gave a moderate temperature and these are inhabited by *men* and *birds* and herds of *wild beasts*.

Clouds, rain, winds

He added clouds to the sky so that they might furnish sudden showers to make the fruits of the trees and of the ground grow with their gentle sprinkling. With the help of the sun these are filled like water skins from the rivers by a hidden law, and then, rising through the upper air, they pour out the water they have taken up, driven by the force of the winds. From them come rainstorms, snow, and round hail when the cold damp wind breathes out its blasts which, penetrating the clouds, drive out the streams just as they make them. Each of

the winds takes to itself a nature of its own from its
proximity to the zone where it is born.

Orders of spirits

Beyond the firmament in which He fixed the shining stars He
placed the *ethereal heaven* and gave it as a habitation to
troops of *angels* whom the worthy contemplation and
marvellous sweetness of God refresh throughout the ages.
This also He adorned with stars and the *shining sun*, laying
down the law, by which a star should run within fixed limits
through the part of heaven entrusted to it.

He afterwards placed beneath this the *airy heavens*,
shining with the lunary body, which throughout their high
places abound in troops of *spirits* who sympathize or rejoice
with us as things go well or ill. They are accustomed to carry
the prayers of men through the air and to beseech God to
have mercy on them, and to bring back intimations of God's
will, either in dreams or by voice or by other signs, through
doing which they become wise.

The space below the moon abounds in evil *demons*, who
are skilled to cheat and deceive and tempt us; often they
assume a body made of air and appear to us and many things
often follow. They even hold intercourse with women and
make them pregnant, generating in an unholy manner. So
therefore He made the heavens to be inhabited by *three
orders of spirits* that each one might look out for something
and renew the world from the renewed seed of things.

The sea

The sea too He distinguished by various forms that from
itself it might produce the forms of things, generating
throughout the ages. Indeed, part of it burns and part freezes
and the third part, getting a moderate temperature from the
other two, ministers to our needs.

That part which burns surrounds a gulf and fierce people,

and its divers streams, flowing back, separate this from the orb of earth, increasing fire from fire. Thither descend those who transgress the laws and reject God; whither their perverse will leads them they go, eager to destroy what is forbidden to them. There stands the stern-eyed judge holding his equal balance and giving to each one his merits and his deserts.

The second part, which freezes, rolls about the foreshorn sands which it is the first to generate from the near-by vapor when it is mingled with the rays of Venus's star. This star, the Arabs say, makes shining gems when it passes through the Fishes while its waters look back at the flames. These gems by their virtues benefit the people who wear them, and make many well and keep them so. These too the Maker distinguished by their kinds as He did all things, that we might discern from their forms and from their colors of what kinds they are and of what manifest virtues.

The third form of the sea which circles our orb furnishes us many good things owing to its proximity. For it nourishes fishes and produces salt in abundance, and bears back and forth ships carrying our commerce, by the profits of which the poor man becomes suddenly rich. It makes fertile the neighboring soil and feeds the birds who, they say, are generated from it along with the fishes and, although unlike, are moved by the laws of nature. The sea is dominated by them more than by the fishes, and they fly lightly up from it through space and seek the lofty regions. But its moisture drives the fishes beneath the waves and keeps them there, and does not permit them to live when they get out into the dry light. These too the Maker distinguished according to their species and to the different ones gave each his nature, whence through the ages they were to become admirable and healthful to the sick.

Fish

For men say that the *barbel* restrains the heat of passion but makes blind those who eat it often. The *thymallus*, which has

its name from the flower thyme, smells so that it betrays the
fish that often eat of it until all the fishes in the river smell
like itself. They say that the *muraenas*, contrary to all laws,
are all the feminine sex, yet they copulate and reproduce and
multiply their offspring from a different kind of seed. For
often snakes come together along the shore where they are,
and they make the sound of pleasing hissing and, calling out
the muraenas, join with them according to custom. It is also
remarkable that the *remora*, half a foot long, holds fast the
ship to which it adheres at sea just as though it were fast
aground, and does not permit the vessel to move until it lets
go; because of this power it is to be feared. And that which
they call the *swordfish*, because it does injury with its sharp
beak, people often fear to approach with a ship when it is
swimming, for if it is captured it at once makes a hole in the
vessel, cuts it in pieces, and sinks it suddenly in a whirlpool.
The *serra* makes itself feared by ships because of its crest; it
fixes to them as it swims underneath, cuts them to pieces
and throws the pieces into the waves, wherefore its crest is
to be feared like a sword. And the *water dragon*, which
men say has poison under its wings, is to be feared by those
who capture it; whenever it strikes it does harm by pouring
out its poison. The *torpedo* is said to have another kind
of destruction, for if any one touches it when it is alive,
straightway his arms and his feet grow torpid and so do
his other members and they lose their functions just as
though they were dead, so harmful is the emanation of its
body.

Islands

To those and the other fishes God gave the sea, and He
added to it many realms among the waves, which men
inhabit and which are renowned because of the fertility
which the earth produces there from its fruitful soil.

Of these *Britain* is said to be the foremost and best,
producing in its fruitfulness every single thing. For it bears

crops which throughout the year give the noble gifts of fragrance for the use of man, and it has woods and glades with honey dripping in them, and lofty mountains and broad green fields, fountains and rivers, fishes and cattle and wild beasts, fruit trees, gems, precious metals, and whatever creative nature is in the habit of furnishing.

Besides all these it has fountains healthful because of their hot waters which nourish the sick and provide pleasing baths, which quickly send people away cured with their sickness driven out. So *Bladud* established them when he held the scepter of the kingdom, and he gave them the name of his consort *Alaron*. These are of value to many sick because of the healing of their water, but most of all to women, as often the water has demonstrated.

Near to this island lies *Thanet* which abounds in many things but lacks the death-dealing serpent, and if any of its earth is drunk mixed with wine it takes away poison. Our ocean also divides the *Orkneys* from us. These are divided into thirty-three islands by the sundering flood; twenty lack cultivation and the others are cultivated. *Thule* receives its name "furthest" from the sun, because of the solstice which the summer sun makes there, turning its rays and shining no further, and taking away the day, so that always throughout the long night the air is full of shadows, and making ice congealed by the benumbing cold, which prevents the passage of ships.

The most outstanding island after our own is said to be *Ireland* with its happy fertility. It is larger and produces no bees, and no birds except rarely, and it does not permit snakes to breed in it. Whence it happens that if earth or a stone is carried away from there and added to any other place it drives away snakes and bees. The island of *Gades* lies next to *Herculean Gades*, and there grows there a tree from whose bark a gum drips out of which gems are made, breaking all laws.

The *Hesperides* are said to contains a watchful dragon who, men say, guards the golden apples under the leaves. The *Gorgades* are inhabited by women with goats' bodies

who are said to surpass hares in the swiftness of their
running. *Argyre* and *Chryse* bear, it is said, gold and silver
just as Corinth does common stones. *Ceylon* blooms
pleasantly because of its fruitful soil, for it produces two
crops in a single year; twice it is summer, twice spring, twice
men gather grapes and other fruits, and it is also most
pleasing because of its shining gems. *Tiles* produces flowers
and fruits in an eternal spring, green throughout the seasons.

The Otherworld

The island of apples which men call *"The Fortunate Isle"*
gets its name from the fact that it produces all things of
itself; the fields there have no need of the ploughs of the
farmers and all cultivation is lacking except what nature
provides. Of its own accord it produces grain and grapes,
and apple trees grow in its woods from the close-clipped
grass. The ground of its own accord produces everything
instead of merely grass, and people live there a hundred years
or more.

There nine sisters rule by a pleasing set of laws those who
come to them from our country. She who is first of them is
more skilled in the healing art, and excels her sisters in the
beauty of her person. *Morgen* is her name, and she has
learned what useful properties all the herbs contain, so that
she can cure sick bodies. She also knows an art by which to
change her shape, and to cleave the air on new wings like
Daedalus; when she wishes she is at Brest, Chartres, or Pavia,
and when she wills she slips down from the air onto your
shores.

And men say that she has taught mathematics to her
sisters, Moronoe, Mazoe, Gliten, Glitonea, Gliton, Tyronoe,
Thitis, Thitis best known for her cither. Thither after the
battle of Camlan we took the wounded Arthur, guided by
Barinthus to whom the waters and the stars of heaven were
well known. With him steering the ship we arrived there with
the prince, Morgen received us with fitting honor, and in her

chamber she placed the king on a golden bed and with her own hand she uncovered his honorable wound and gazed at it for a long time. At length she said that health could be restored to him if he stayed with her for a long time and made use of her healing art. Rejoicing, therefore, we entrusted the king to her and returning spread our sails to the favoring winds.'

THE CREATION OF THE WORLD

The increasingly firm statements regarding the dichotomy between the mystical and material life are not Christian dogma. As soon as Ganieda has taken to the woods, we have a new wisdom poem presented to us, from the mouth of the bard Taliesin as inspired by Minerva. In this remarkable sequence which stretches from the starry realms through the natural orders of life into the UnderWorld, the apparently opposed modes of life, mystical and material, are resolved; they are demonstrated as a unity in which the lesser world reflects and partakes of the greater.

The sequence is an exposition taking the form of a cosmic model which has many details in common with classical sources,[1] but also contains quite independent and probably Celtic or originally Druidic symbolism.[2] Before going into this lesson in both metaphysics, physics, and biology, we should summarise its position in the overall progress of Merlin around the Wheel of Life. The Creation of the World or Worlds is not idly placed at this point in the *Vita*, it appears to be prompted by the question that Merlin poses: 'What is the nature of wind and rainstorms?' But it deals with much more than weather lore, and eventually brings us to the potent subject of miraculous springs or fountains, so leading to Merlin's final cure.

This query about the weather is heard at the beginning of Merlin's mystical and seasonal journey, when he asks 'How does it happen that the seasons are not all the same?'[3] When the question first arises, he is raging against the natural cycle of the seasons in his madness, but by the time Taliesin has appeared Merlin has gone through the following stages:

1 Intolerable grief and guilt leading to madness.
2 Living as a wild man in the wood, reaching the hilltop fountain.
3 Returning to human society through the power of music.
4 Attempting to resolve problems relating to sexuality or sensuality.
5 Onset of prophetic or far-sight.
6 Sacrificial theme of Threefold Death.
7 Flight to woods again, with increased perceptions.
8 Lord of the Animals, death of surrogate husband rival.
9 Return to human society as captive: allegory of human existence in form of doorkeeper and hopeful youth.
10 Reasoned return to woods, building of observatory.
11 Prophetic history uttered through star gazing.
12 Reasoned posing of the season question: what is the nature of weather? (See Figures 4, 6, and 8.)

This cyclical pattern, in which Merlin travels back and forward between madness and sanity, the wildwood and civilisation, primal unpolarised energy and sexual polarity, ignorance and wisdom, is one in which the clarity and intensity of the power of consciousness increases and simultaneously becomes balanced and expressed. The balancing power is in the form of his sister, Ganieda.

Only after undergoing the spiralling changes that appear through interaction can Merlin be ready to ask the question in a balanced manner, and to receive a balanced answer. He is in the position of the initiate in the ancient Mysteries, which formalised the roles that apply to any man or woman during the inner transformations of the psyche which are inseparable from spiritual growth.

Merlin has experienced fervour, frenzy, far-sight, and future-sight. He is now ready for a more mature teaching, one in which the elements of the natural world are shown to be at one with the elements of the supernatural world. He has experienced the expanded consciousness, and now he integrates its power within a reasoned framework.

It must be stressed that this 'reasoned framework' is a far cry from materialist reason or logic; it is still a mystical and religious wonder-filled vision. But it also carries a model of conscious life and its myriad forms, a model which helps the initiate or mystic to establish relationships which enable him or her to return to the outer world and serve within it.

The Creation of The World is divided into a number of coherent sections, commencing with the divine macrocosm or greater universe, and concluding beyond the natural world. Various other spiritual, angelic and demonic realms are also located spatially and metaphysically within the system. The sub-divisions of the creation poem are as follows:

1 four primary elements of creation out of nothing
2 the starry heavens
3 the air (atmosphere or sky)
4 the sea
5 the earth, which in turn is divided into five parts, reflecting the fivefold division of the greater World in which it stands:
   i middle: extreme heat
   ii outer zone (a): extreme cold (North Pole)
   iii outer zone (b): extreme cold (South Pole)
   iv temperate zone (a)
   v temperate zone (b).

It is in the last two zones where men, birds, and animals live. Having descended through Origination, Starry Heaven, Sky, Earth, the sequence then repeats the pattern giving more details of each zone. The formal educational structure is clear; the pattern is defined in short, then the details of each defined area are amplified. Similar patterns are still found in traditional songs to the present day, where a group of numerical songs (The 'Keys of Heaven')[4] present an ordered descent from divine origination through to the material world. Symbolism of this type was embedded deeply into the communal imagination, and was not only the product of the learned scholars or travelling bards and poets (see Figures 9 and 10).

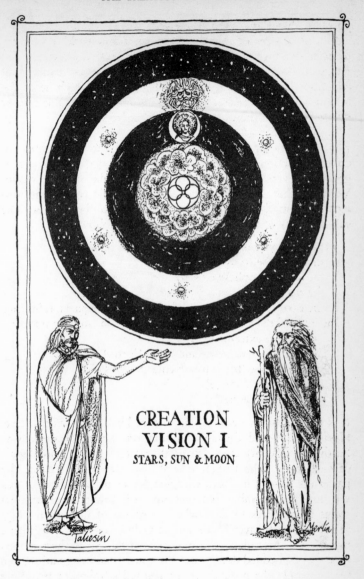

Figure 9 *Creation vision: stars/sun/moon*

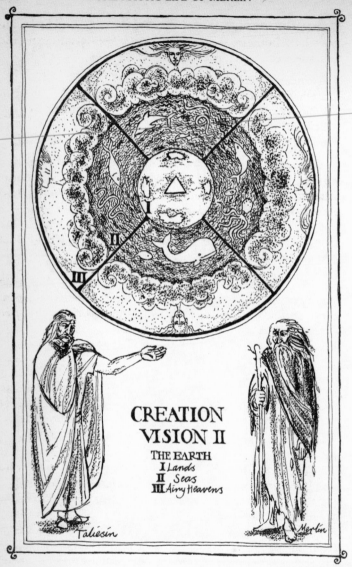

Figure 10 *Creation vision: the earth*

After defining the origin of rainstorms, snow, and hail within the winds born in the various zones, the stellar exposition recommences:

1 firmament (fixed bright stars)
2 ethereal heaven (angels, the sun, moving stars)
3 higher airy heaven (the moon, spirits sympathetic to mankind)
4 lower airy heaven (below the moon, deceptive demons).

Three orders of spirits are defined to operate the universe: *angelic, sympathetic, deceptive*. We might add that in the usual esoteric and religious traditions, the first zone of fixed bright stars is often termed arch-angelic.

The sea brings us back to the earthly zones, and is divided into three parts:

1 Hot, leading to hell or the realm of Judgement. This image is of ancient origin, and reflects not only orthodox religious belief of the medieval period, but has its roots in both Celtic and Classical mythology.[5]
2 Cold, creates jewels or crystals with varying powers.
3 Moderate, bringing the benefits of life.

There follows a detailed discourse on the *biology* of the sea, most of which was customary for writers of the period. The exposition is now being opened out; from primary origins it has gradually unfolded and now encompasses *geography*.

The geography is more specifically Celtic-British, and praises Britain as the most fruitful of lands. From fertility of land, we move to the springs that water the land, and then on to islands that surround the land.

This triple progression is suggestive of the Celtic Otherworld; from the mainland, through a sacred spring or well, to the magical islands or Otherworld. The islands listed are mainly classical in origin, but set the scene for the presentation of the *Island of Apples* or the *Fortunate Island*. We have arrived at

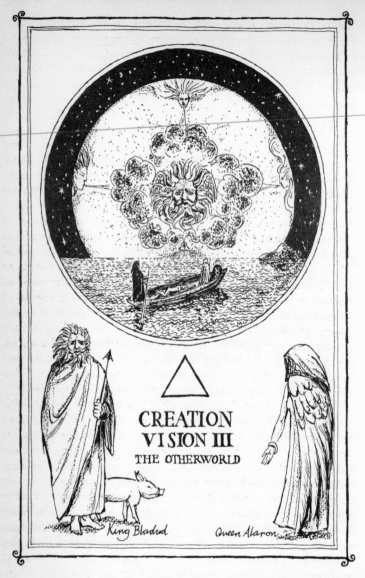

Figure 11 *Creation vision: the Otherworld*

last in the realm of the magical Otherworld (see Figure 11).

This section of the Creation poem, perhaps derived from an independent traditional source, is primarily Celtic in its origins and symbols. If we follow the direction of the overall creation model, it leads us in a very clearly defined sequence: stars, sky, sea, lands (Britain and Islands). In Britain, wells and springs preface a series of legendary classical islands, which lead up to the Island of Apples and the myth of Morgen.

There is some significance in the naming of King Bladud and his consort Alaron prior to the introduction of the Celtic Blessed or Fortunate Island and the magical image of Morgen. Bladud, first mentioned in *The History*, was a legendary British king with many attributes close to those of a solar deity. Geoffrey linked Bladud with Appollo, and drew upon a tradition in which (in some variants) the youthful king was cured of a wasting disease by the guidance of a totem animal (the pig) to a hot healing spring. Bladud later built a temple in this place, dedicated to Minerva, and taught the arts of necromancy through the land. He is a typical combination of magical god-image, and sacred king or priest representing the pagan, Druidic system of worship and wisdom. He is, in fact, the tutelary being of the gateway to the Other or UnderWorld, for he initiated the healing springs as a formal therapeutic and worship site. Wells and springs were central to the Celtic culture, having enormous magical and religious significance.

The name Bladud is possibly derived from two Celtic language words, *Bel* and *dydd* or possibly *derwdd*. It means literally 'bright/dark' or bright priest. A similar image is encountered in *The Prophecies* where the god Janus guards the gateway to the Otherworld; Janus was a twofold being looking both into light and darkness, the keeper of all doorways. In both cases the tutelary figure precedes the appearance of a primal Goddess image; in *The Prophecies* he is associated with Ariadne who ends the solar cycle, while in the *Vita* Morgen appears with her nine sisters as ruler of the Otherworld. The similarities between these two images suggest a common tradition, one which is found in a number of other tales, songs, and associated themes dealing with the passage from the human world to the Other or Underworld.[6]

The descent of the Creation is therefore: stars/sky/sea/the land/wells and springs with guardian power/magical islands/ the realm of Morgen and her nine sisters. It is a typical Celtic motif that we pass *through* the well or spring to reach the magical realms of primal potency, though this is only implied in Geoffrey's sequence and not fully stated.

The mixture of classical material from current sources available to Geoffrey with native mythological or legendary persons and themes prevents us from seeking after a presumed 'original', as no original in the literary sense may be found due to the dream-like oral preservation of the British images and story sequences.

The image of a goddess and nine sisters is found widespread throughout world mythology, though the number of sisters or aspects varies. Geoffrey is restating a theme already found in the Welsh poem *The Spoils of Annwm*, which possibly predates the *Vita* where Arthur seeks a magical cauldron attended by nine maidens.[7] Morgen's knowledge of therapy and her magical flight are all attributes of a goddess.[8]

Arthur must remain in this land for a long time, while Morgen undertakes his cure; this is one of the earliest references to the golden bed which would soon play such an important part in the Grail symbolism, where wounded king, bed, and the sanctity of the land are indissolubly linked together. If the king is healed, the land is healed.

It is this therapeutic motif which makes Geoffrey's account unique, setting the tone for a mass of subsequent literature. In psychological terms it is the traditional image of inner healing, which is in the noble hand of the feminine aspects of consciousness. In ancient culture these aspects or modes were deified, and such divinity still resonates about the figure of Morgen, mistress of flight, astrology, therapy and shape-changing. These magical arts are the abilities not only of pagan deities, but which are constantly attributed to the Druidic faith and practices.

Through this section of lyrical magical reminiscence, the two separate 'lives' of Merlin (Merlin Ambrosius who predicted before King Vortigern, and Merlin Celidonius who fled mad into the woods) are contrived to meet together. Arthur waits in a timeless fruitful land until the goddess has healed him.

The connection between a magically gifted woman, a goddess, and the theme of healing are stated also in *The Prophecies*, where a maiden purifies three springs of Life, Desire, and Death, and so becomes a mature goddess uniting the land of Britain, holding the towers of London and the forests of Scotland in either hand.[9]

As the king is the focal point, the human emblem of the power of the land, it is to the goddess Morgen that the wounded Arthur is carried after the battle of Camlann.

The pseudo-historical action is deliberately split into two parts, for we have the mythic conclusion to Arthur's last battle, then the historical sequence up to and including the battle in the form of a retrospective utterance based upon a mixture of *The Prophecies* and the general chronicled events found in *The History*.[10]

It is typical of Geoffrey's flair for poetry and drama that the most memorable and moving scene is given as the keystone to the entire myth of Arthur; his kingship, his battles with the Saxons, his betrayal by Modred are all subsidiary to the simple motif of his fatal and enduring wound, the long term of healing in a magical eternal land, and the care of a goddess.

In magical or psychological images, it is the highly lit and moving scene of the wounded king being carried over the sea and coming to rest upon a golden bed; he is waiting, and will come again. We feel this intuitively, and the longing for the return of the king is expressed in very practical terms by Taliesin: 'Then the people should send someone to tell the chief to come back in a swift ship if he has recovered his strength, that he may drive off the enemy with his accustomed vigour and establish the citizens in their former peace.'

But Merlin declares that it is the will of the highest Judge that the Britons shall lose their noble kingdom for a long time. Out of the glow of the myth, we find a tone of Celtic nationalism creeping into the narrative, a feature prominent in *The Prophecies* but hitherto unstated. The magical and mythical theme of Arthur has prompted a restatement of the nationalistic sentiments found in a number of British/Welsh poems.

Before moving on to this more prosaic but still mythical sequence of pseudo-history, in which the remainder of the Arthur legend is recounted, there is one interesting character who must be discussed: *Barinthus*, 'to whom the waters and the stars of heaven were well known'. There are several likely characters who relate to Barinthus, not the least being the god Bran who waded across the sea to Ireland and made a bridge of himself; or Barrintus who sailed to a magical island in the *Life of Brendan*.[11] But the linguistic or literary sources are merely evidence of the existence of a primal image: the Ferryman. He is the power of safe passage, of transit from world to world. The classical image is that of Charon, ferryman of the river Styx, but the figure transcends all names and cultures. In folk tradition as late as the twentieth century, this figure, originally a sea-god and star-guide, is found actively represented in song and ritual. In the *Dilly Song* or *Keys of Heaven*, a verse appears: 'Six is the Ferryman in the boat that o'er the river floats-oh', where six plays an important transitional role in a sequence reaching from the stellar heavens to the kingdom of earth. This sequence seems to have close relationship to the mystical Tree of Life that appeared in medieval Europe from Jewish or Arabic sources grafted onto a native cosmic-tree tradition. In the *Padstow May Song*, it is Saint George who is 'out on the salt sea' in his long boat, during a crucial scene in the dance-drama in which death and resurrection are portrayed. In the broader Arthurian traditions that developed shortly after Geoffrey, mysterious barges and boats proliferate; but Barinthus was the first sailor across that mysterious sea lit by stars.[12]

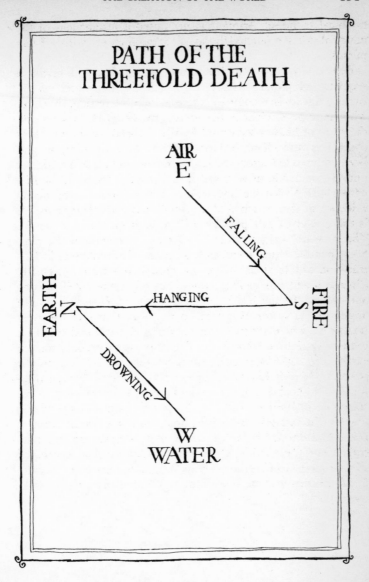

PATH OF THE THREEFOLD DEATH

AIR
E

FALLING

EARTH
N

HANGING

FIRE
S

DROWNING

W
WATER

Figure 12 *Path of the Threefold Death and the elements*

CHAPTER 11
I Merlin remembers
II The Three Faces of Merlin

The Heavens in stead of water bloud shall showre,
And famine shall both young and old devour,
Droop and be sad shall the *Red dragon* then,
But after mickle time be blithe agen.

Thomas Heywood, Merlin, 1641.

Merlin is restored to a full memory by the long mystical and metaphysical exposition; he supports it by a historical set of incidents from the arrival of the Saxons to the rise and fall of King Arthur's realm. This historical sequence brings us the factual support for the preceding myth of Arthur (Chapter 10), and leads the reader towards a key motif: Merlin's lengthy experience of the land and its inhabitants.

MERLIN REMEMBERS

The narrative of the *Vita* is once again filled out with 'evidence'; Merlin enters into a detailed set of memories, which are actually a chronological/historical passage drawn mainly from Geoffrey's *History*. This passage does not contain material directly pertinent to the mystical life or inner growth of Merlin; it is used to corroborate the mythical sequence dealing with Arthur that closes the Creation of the World.

We should see this material, as with other self-referring or pseudo-historical prophecies in the *Vita*, as being essential aspects of Geoffrey's artistic reassembly of traditional lore; he does not hesitate to draw upon his own earlier work, *The History*, as this would have been familiar to many if not all of his noble listeners.[1]

During the 'memoires' of early campaigns and treacheries, two subjects which are intertwined with the magical and psychological implications of the *Vita* are touched upon: Arthur's betrayal by Modred (which led to the final battle and Arthur's 'honourable wound'), and Merlin's great age, a theme which is expanded shortly in a separate passage which embodies a Celtic tradition.

But the placing of the historical sequence as an ethnocentric corroboration of the cosmological and geocentric teaching has a more subtle role. Merlin is able to recall in great detail the historical events during his life; and now, following the creative world-picture, he is clearly regaining his senses.

The question 'What causes the weather?' or 'What is the nature of the wheel or cycle of changes?' has been answered in the most comprehensive manner by the learned Taliesin; Merlin finds that this answer corresponds to his own detailed experience of life. He has gained a balance between his grief and the resulting madness, and the overview or cosmic view, with its harmonic results that affect not only the homeland and the individual, but reach through into the magically potent Otherworld where true healing dwells in the form of a goddess.

So Merlin's return to sanity is not merely a reversal back to his prior state of kingship, for too many deep and enduring changes have arisen for this to be so. But he can grasp and utter the link between the Fourfold Cycle that results in all creation, and the expressed cycle of human sorrows, rises, falls, and joys. No one has seen so many savage battles as Merlin, says Taliesin, and Merlin agrees, stating his own long life as proof of this harrowing truth.

We are beginning to meet the Merlin best known to later popular traditions: the old man who represents knowledge and wisdom through long experience.

THE THREE FACES OF MERLIN

Merlin appears in three ways in the work of Geoffrey:

1 a youth who utters *The Prophecies*;
2 a mature man who is involved with kingship or is a king himself, but later renounces such matters through a madness brought on by grief;
3 a very wise old man who eventually retires to lead a wholly spiritual life.

In the many studies of Merlin that have been made, it is almost customary for commentators to say that Geoffrey has combined two separate traditions (Merlin of *The Prophecies* and Merlin of the madness found in the *Vita*). While these themes are apparently derived from Wales and Scotland, where similar tales are known from manuscript and tradition, very little attention has been paid to the concept that they might separately represent fragments of one diffuse but coherent tradition. Geoffrey certainly attempted to merge both branches together, but this does not ultimately mean that their union is only due to his intellect, or that they were utterly separate prior to Geoffrey's assembly.

The Three Faces of Merlin, which are of course the three aspects of human psychic growth and physical growth, are a direct parallel to the three aspects of the Goddess (maiden, mature woman, crone). Triple symbolism through specific personalities is also found in the Grail legends which blossomed shortly after Geoffrey dealt with his themes. The three Grail Achievers, Galahad, Perceval, and Bors, are an example which bears some relationship to the triple presentations of Merlin in Geoffrey's work, which was drawn from tradition.[2]

We can find such interconnection in many tales and ballads from oral tradition, in which characters reappear in quite separate narratives, yet are clearly interconnected in ways shown by their behaviour, their symbolic attributes, and their persistence through time in the common imagination. The same might be said of Merlin; his full story is a triplicity, the sources may be separate, but the sum is a unity.

Geoffrey clearly felt this to be true, thus pre-empting the

modern study of the psyche by at least seven centuries, presenting a proto-psychology which still holds good today. But this proto-psychology is the result of the wisdom teachings of early cultures, not the intellectual invention of one man or group of men.

It would be foolish to suggest that Geoffrey 'knew what he was doing' in terms of modern psychology; but the myriad sources that embodied the old traditions knew collectively, drawing upon persons, motifs and symbols which percolated through the medium of firstly a pagan and then a Christian culture without radical change. When this lore became encapsulated in the Grail legends, which were outside the orthodox Church, they were not suppressed or challenged; and they changed the face of Western literature and history through their influence.

Finally it is worth stating the obvious: there are not two traditions of Merlin (Merlin Emrys and Merlin the Wild Man), but three; Geoffrey has conflated the last two in the *Vita*, where Merlin appears firstly, as a mature king with a lush sensual wife and secondly as an incredibly ancient man who has seen all things come to pass. The first tradition, that of the youth who is partly human and partly divine or superhuman, is found in *The Prophecies*, but this tradition also leaps to the very end of time.

Merlin, therefore, is possessed of all the ages and sorrows of the human race while still a youth. The verses of *The Prophecies* show this very clearly indeed, not only carrying future history but the apocalytic vision of the end of time, in which the creation of the solar system is withdrawn by a goddess, leaving only four winds to blast against one another. These are the same four that Taliesin cites as the first causes of all creation, in the *Vita*.

The subject of Merlin's great age is dealt with in our text chapter, but the three traditions referred to above, which are really three phases of one tradition, faintly remind us of a primal legend: Merlin is the First and Last Man.

CHAPTER 12

I *The healing fountain*
II *Merlin's prayer*
III *Merlin's great age*

'In water there is a quality endowed with a blessing,
On God it is most just to meditate aright;
To God it is proper to supplicate with seriousness,
Since no obstacle can there be to obtain a reward from him.
Three times have I been born, I know by meditation;
It would be miserable for a person not to come
And gain all science of the world collected in my breast,
For I know what has been, what in future will occur . . .'
          The Song of Taliesin (trans. Lady C. Guest).

A healing fountain breaks out at the foot of the mountains, and
bathing in its waters finally restores Merlin utterly to health
and sanity. He offers up a prayer thanking divinity for the gift
of healing, and asks yet another vital question, 'Whence comes
this virtue?'. Taliesin again obliges by a further wisdom
sequence on fountains, rivers, and lakes. Princes and chieftains
assemble to bid Merlin take up his kingdom once again, but he
states that his incredible age debars him from such activities,
and that he intends to withdraw into spiritual contemplation.

THE HEALING FOUNTAIN

While he was speaking thus the servants hurried in and

announced to him that a new fountain had broken out at the
foot of the mountains and was pouring out pure waters
which were running through all the hollow valley and
swirling through the fields as they slipped along. Both
therefore quickly rose to see the new fountain, and having
seen it Merlin sat down again on the grass and praised the
spot and the flowing waters, and marvelled that they had
come out of the ground in such a fashion. Soon afterward,
becoming thirsty, he leaned down to the stream and drank
freely and bathed his temples in its waves, so that the water
passed through the passages of his bowels and stomach,
settling the vapors within him, and at once he regained his
reason and knew himself, and all his madness departed and
the sense which had long remained torpid in him revived,
and he remained what he had once been – sane and intact
with his reason restored. Therefore, praising God, he turned
his face toward the stars and uttered devout words of praise.
'O King, through whom the order of the starry heavens
exists, through whom the sea and the land with its pleasing
grass give forth and nourish their offspring and with their
profuse fertility give frequent aid to mankind, through whom
sense has returned and the error of my mind has vanished! I
was carried away from myself and like a spirit I knew the
acts of past peoples and predicted the future. Then since I
knew the secrets of things and the flight of birds and the
wandering motions of the stars and the gliding of the fishes,
all this vexed me and denied a natural rest to my human
mind by a severe law. Now I have come to myself and I seem
to be moved with a vigor such as was wont to animate my
limbs. Therefore, highest father, ought I to be obedient to
thee, that I may show forth thy most worthy praise from a
worthy heart, always joyfully making joyful offerings. For
twice thy generous hand has benefitted me alone, in giving
me the gift of this new fountain out of the green grass. For
now I have the water which hitherto I lacked, and by
drinking of it my brains have been made whole. But whence
comes this virtue, O dear companion, that this new fountain
breaks out thus, and makes me myself again who up to now

was as though insane and beside myself?'

Taliesin answered, 'The opulent Regulator of things divided the rivers according to their kinds, and added moreover to each a power of its own, that they might often prove of benefit to the sick. For there are fountains and rivers and lakes throughout the world which by their power cure many, and often do so.

At Rome, for instance, flows swift *Albula*, with its healthgiving stream which men say cures wounds with its sure healing. There is another fountain, called *Cicero's*, which flows in Italy, which cures the eyes of all injuries. The *Ethiopians* also are said to have a pool which makes a face on which it is poured shine just as though from oil. Africa has a fountain, commonly called *Zama*, a drink from it produces melodious voices by its sudden power. Lake *Clitorius* in Italy gives a distaste for wine; those who drink from the fountain of *Chios* are said to become dull. The land of *Boeotia* is said to have two fountains; the one makes the drinkers forgetful, the other makes them remember. The same country contains a lake so harmful with its dire plague that it generates madness and the heat of too much passion.

The fountain of *Cyzicus* drives away lust and the love of Venus. In the region of *Campania* there flow, it is said, rivers which when drunk of make the barren fruitful, and the same ones are said to take away madness from men. The land of the *Ethiopians* contains a fountain with a red stream; whoever drinks of this will come back demented. The fountain of *Leinus* never permits miscarriages. There are two fountains in *Sicily*, one of which makes girls sterile and the other makes them fruitful by its kindly law. There are two rivers in *Thessaly* of the greatest power; a sheep drinking of one turns black and is made white by the other, and any one drinking of both spends its life with a variegated fleece.

There is a lake called *Clitumnus* in the Umbrian land which is said at times to produce large oxen, and in the *Reatine Swamp* the hooves of horses become hard as soon as they cross its sands. In the *Asphalt Lake* of Judaea bodies can never sink while life animates them, but on the other hand the land of India has a pool called *Sida* in which nothing floats but sinks at once to the bottom. And there is a *Lake Aloe* in which nothing sinks but all things float even if they are pieces of lead. The fountain of *Marsida* also compels stones to float.

The *River Styx* flows from a rock and kills those who drink of it; the land of Arcadia bears testimony to this form of destruction. The fountain of *Idumea*, changing four times throughout the days, is said to vary its color by a strange rule; for it becomes muddy, then green, then the order changes and it turns red and then becomes clear with a beautiful stream. It is said to retain each one of these colors for three months as the years roll around. There is also a Lake *Trogdytus* whose waves flow out, three times in the day bitter, and three times sweet with a pleasant taste. From a fountain of *Epirus* torches are said to be lighted, and if extinguished to resume their light again. The fountain of the *Garamantes* is said to be so cold in the day time, and on the other hand so hot all night, that it forbids approach on account of its cold or its heat.

There are also hot waters that threaten many because of the heat which they get when they flow through alum or sulphur which have a fiery power, pleasant for healing. God endowed the rivers with these powers and others so that they might be the means of quick healing for the sick, and so that they might make manifest with what power the Creator stands eminent among things while He works thus in them. I think that these waters are healthful in the highest degree and I think that they could afford a quick cure through the water that has thus broken out. They have up to now been flowing about through the dark hollows under the earth like many others that are said to trickle underground. Perhaps their breaking out is due to an obstacle getting in their way, or to the slipping of a stone or a mass of earth. I think that, in making their way back again, they have gradually penetrated the ground and have given us this fountain. You see many such flow along and return again under ground and regain their caverns.'

THE HEALING FOUNTAIN

We now come to the final healing of Merlin's imbalance; the symbol of the curative spring or fountain is met once more. When Merlin made his first temporary recovery from madness, he was found at the top of a mountain, sitting by a spring which was surrounded by nut trees. From this location, he was soothed by the power of music, and made his first return to the world of mortal men.

After the lengthy exposition in which the healing powers of springs in Britain are extolled, with special mention of King Bladud, the guardian figure of the sacred springs of Caer Baddon (Bath, Aquae Sulis), it is not surprising that Merlin is cured by a miraculous spring which breaks out 'at the foot of the mountains'. But we have not been set in readiness for this motif through a merely literary contrivance; springs and fountains are an essential of Celtic transformative lore and magical interaction.[1] In *The Prophecies* a powerful vision of the purification and transformation of the land of Britain is found, in which a goddess acts as the mediating power to change transient energies into permanent balanced power. The ancient Celts had vested such power in the springs and lakes of Gaul that the Roman Empire auctioned them to the highest bidder; each sacred spring or source was full of offerings of immense value in gold, silver, or workmanship.

By the fifth century through to the twelfth century when Geoffrey wrote, such pagan practices had become modified into the worship of saints who patronised springs and wells, with offerings held in churches or great abbeys, and folk customs of throwing small tokens or tying coloured strips of cloth upon the trees at wells.[2] But the oral and popular traditions regarding springs were still very strong, and underwent a potent poetical reinforcement with the appearance of the Grail legends. The tradition of a curative spring, therefore, may be traced back to the earliest records of British or Celtic belief. In modern psychological terms, as in the ancient magical and spiritual systems, the wellspring is the source of energy within the human entity; it is life itself.

Merlin's final cure is revealing not only in its use of an enduring and effective symbol of inner therapy and purification, but in its descriptive details, set in the words of Merlin himself. The content of his thankful prayer is worth examining in detail.

MERLIN'S PRAYER

1 Merlin turns his face to the stars, and praises God the creator; the language is directly derived from the cosmic model uttered by Taliesin during his instruction in reply to the mystical question about the origin of Weather.

2 He describes his subjective experiences as a mad prophet:
  (a) Carried away from himself (i.e. not self-conscious).
  (b) Like a spirit, knowing the acts of past peoples and predicting the future. Merlin's consciousness has separated from the regular time-stream which establishes self-awareness. He is therefore able to see both past and future. It is significant that Geoffrey or his source describes the knowledge of past peoples, which is termed 'necromancy' in connection with King Bladud (*The History*), as this knowledge forms one of the hallowed aspects of a heightened awareness through the magical traditions. The same detailed description applies to knowledge of the future, though this is a more commonplace theme.[3]
  c The *motion* of his transcendent awareness (flight of birds, gliding of fish, movement of stars) denied Merlin his natural rest. His mind was strained beyond normal endurance, and so he became unbalanced.

3 God has blessed him with a fountain from within the green grass or earth, which purifies his consciousness, and restores his vigour. The framework, as we have seen, of Merlin's restoration is in the shape of
  (a) personal maturity through human relationships and sexual polarity, and

(b) through cosmology, in the form of a spiritual education in answer to mystical questions first posed on a human level, but later moving to higher realms of consciousness, gaining a new level of answer with each transformation or change of mode. The culmination of this cure is in the form of a blessing, an act of grace, but this power has obviously been flowing ready to meet Merlin, as we discover from the next detailed exposition of Taliesin.

The healing waters of the world

Merlin now asks 'Whence comes this virtue?', and we are launched into yet another teaching poem of the bards, mixed copiously with classical allusion. The drift of this is to act, once again, as 'proof' of the curative properties of fountains, rivers, and lakes; it also gives a highly entertaining and curious speech for the listener avid to imbibe ancient wisdom. The majority of the sources listed are from classical or neo-classical texts, but one or two demand further comment, as they demonstrate yet again the importance of polarity in traditional teachings through story-telling.

These examples of polarity not only follow the general theme which runs through the text of the *Vita*, but also remind us that water sources may curse as well as cure, and that Merlin's cure is due to grace and wisdom, not merely to chance. In a following section of the narrative, we find the motif of poison playing its role, thus setting into place one of the last pieces of the puzzle of the mysterious women in Merlin's life.[4] But first let us consider a few examples of polarity:

Boeotia: a fountain of forgetfulness and one of memory.
Sicily: one of sterility and one of fertility.
Thessaly: a sheep drinking of one turns black, of another, white; drinking of both makes for a variegated sheep. This image of black and white sheep is also found in the tale of *Peredur* in the Mabinogion,[5] and like a number of images of chess, chequers or similar polarity games, represents the

interplay of energies.

Judaea has a lake in which bodies cannot sink, while *India* has a pool called Sida in which nothing floats.

Idumea changes it colours with the seasons: muddy, green, red, and clear, for three months of each year.

Garamantes is alternatively extremely hot and cold.

The alternating images are not left to the chance assumptions of the listeners, their polarity is hammered home by repeated examples. Other properties include driving to madness, preservation, control of lust. There are widespread examples of the Three Fountains found in *The Prophecies*; three primal sources of Life, Desire, and Death.[6]

Taliesin concludes by describing the curative properties of sulphur springs, and the divine direction of curative waters. He then states clearly that the fountain has been 'flowing about through the dark hollows underground . . . in making their way back the waters have gradually penetrated the earth and have given us this fountain'. Here is the classic symbol of energies breaking through into outer cognition, not only an analogy of the psyche, but also of the body. Both derive from an enduring intuition that all life originates *beneath*; the modern 'subconscious' is merely an intellectual restatement of the power known to the ancients as the UnderWorld. But the UnderWorld was far more than a mere vague area of human consciousness, it was the hidden source of all energy, all life, all transformation, all death, both material, biological, psychic, magical, and even spiritual. It is this UnderWorld that is thinly masked by Taliesin's statement.

MERLIN'S GREAT AGE

While they were doing these things a rumor ran all about that a new fountain had broken out in the woods of Celidon, and that drinking from it had cured a man who had for a long time been suffering from madness and had lived in these same woods after the manner of the wild beasts. Soon therefore the princes and the chieftains came to see it and to rejoice with the prophet who had been cured by the water. After they had informed him in detail of the status of his country and had asked him to resume his scepter, and to deal with his people with his accustomed moderation, he said, 'Young men, my time of life, drawing on toward old age, and so possessing my limbs that with my weakened vigor I can scarce pass through the fields, does not ask this of me. I have already lived long enough, rejoicing in happy days while an abundance of great riches smiled profusely upon me.

In that wood there stands an oak in its hoary strength which old age, that consumes everything, has so wasted away that it lacks sap and is decaying inwardly. I saw this when it first began to grow and I even saw the fall of the acorn from which it came, and a woodpecker standing over it and watching the branch. Here I have seen it grow of its own accord, watching it all, and, fearing for it in these fields, I marked the spot with my retentive mind. So you see I have lived a long time and now the weight of age holds me back and I refuse to reign again. When I remain under the green leaves the riches of Calidon delight me more than the gems that India produces, or the gold that Tagus is said to have on its shore, more than the crops of Sicily or the grapes of pleasant Methis, more than lofty turrets or cities girded with high walls or robes fragrant with Tyrian perfumes. Nothing pleases me enough to tear me away from my Calidon which in my opinion is always pleasant. Here shall I remain while I live, content with apples and grasses, and I shall purify my body with pious fastings that I may be worthy to partake of the life everlasting.'

MERLIN'S GREAT AGE

Our next image is of a gathering of princes and chieftains, soliciting Merlin to resume his role of ruler. The traditional theme of the wise elder, consulted by the leaders of the people, is becoming established.

The prophet refuses to return to his throne, and employs a sequence which is very likely to have been a poem in its own right, either attached to Merlin in oral tradition, or to other figures. It concerns the symbol of the *Oldest Creature*, and is found in other Celtic sources. The oldest creature is thought to be the most wise, for he or she has seen all things come to pass; this symbolism is therefore attached to Merlin in this third phase of Wise Old Man.[7]

Once again Geoffrey expands the sequence by adding some poetic touches of his own, such as Merlin's rejection couched in terms of exotic temptations that no longer affect his senses. The text is now beginning to move towards a religious conclusion, for Merlin seeks 'the life everlasting'. In this context, however, we must be aware that his spiritual retreat to the woods is a hallowed way of seeking insight that is found worldwide; it is not limited to Christianity alone, and may equally be an echo of the older Merlin/Wild Man/Wise Man traditions which were essentially pagan and perhaps Druidic.

The tone of Geoffrey's concluding verses is one of resolution; he draws in the various threads of tradition regarding Merlin, insight, prophecy, and spiritual maturity or mystical quest, and synthesises them into a finale that includes pagan and Christian sentiment or wisdom. Indeed, these elements are quite closely fused together in the closing verses of the *Vita*, and it is not possible to separate them for dissection without losing the power and value of the narrative itself. While on one level this may represent the overall salvation of seers in medieval tales, received into the bosom of the Church upon their death (though this does not happen to Merlin), it also represents a deeper insight.

The resolution of the *Vita* shows the union between paganism and Christianity, it merges the ancient wild powers and seership with a deeper spiritual experience symbolised by Merlin's cure and his final withdrawal. We shall return to this theme shortly, for it is a transcendent promise, and not a merely orthodox piece of literary juggling.

CHAPTER 13
A catalogue of birds

After these things shall come forth a Heron from the forest of Calaterium, which shall fly around the island of Britain for two years together. With her nocturnal cry she shall call together the winged kind, and assemble to her all sort of fowls.

The Prophecies of Merlin.

The Eagle said: I have been here for a great period of time, and when I first came hither there was a rock here, from the top of which I pecked at the Stars every evening . . . now it is not so much as a span high.

Kilhwch and Olwen, the *Mabinogion* (trans. Lady C. Guest).

Wisdom is contagious; the newly healed Merlin immediately utters a long discourse upon the type and habits of birds, mainly taken from the encyclopedic books available to the medieval scholar. He knows of birds, he says, through his long period in the woods close to nature. Certain magical symbols from antiquity are found within the passage, which is the second of Three Marvellous Appearances:

1 the Miraculous Spring (Chapter 12)
2 the Flight of Cranes
3 the Madman of the Poisoned Apples (Chapter 14).

A CATALOGUE OF BIRDS

While he was speaking thus, the chiefs caught sight of long lines of cranes in the air, circling through space in a curved

147

line in the shape of certain letters; they could be seen in marshalled squadron in the limpid air. Marvelling at these they asked Merlin to tell why it was that they were flying in such a manner. Merlin presently said to them, 'The Creator of the world gave to the birds as to many other things their proper nature, as I have learned by living in the woods for many days.

'It is therefore the nature of the cranes, as they go through the air, if many are present, that we often see them in their flight form a figure in one way or another. One, by calling, warns them to keep the formation as they fly, lest it break up and depart from the usual figure; when he becomes hoarse another takes his place.'

A CATALOGUE OF BIRDS

Of this list of birds and their rather unusual attributes (which is translated in full in Clarke, 1973), two major symbols are worth comment: the Crane and Woodpecker.

The Crane is linked in early literature with the formation of the letters of the alphabet, originally a magical sequence. In the context of Merlin's narrative career, we may interpret the appearance of cranes in two ways:

1 Classical origins of the Crane and letters: Geoffrey's list is drawn from Isidore, as with earlier items in the *Vita*. The Greeks credited Mercury with the invention of letters, and the crane was a sacred bird to both Mercury and Appollo. In ancient Egyptian culture, the god Thoth bore the head of an Ibis, also associated with letters, learning, and the role of messenger.[1]

2 Possible allusion to the role of messenger: in an earlier scene Merlin is met by a messenger who plays the crwth (cither) or lyre to cure his madness. This Mercurial symbol reminds us that letters were also associated with the traditional seven strings and seven planets. The cranes are a symbol of order read into movement in the skies; they are an

analogy in the natural world of the motions of the stellar world. Their flight marked the changes of the seasons, as does the flight of the Pleiades in the starry heavens.[2]

The Woodpecker appears twice, once as the bird linked to the aged oak that proves Merlin's own long life, and secondly derived from the lists of Isidore, where he pulls nails out of the trees. Classically the relationship between woodpecker and oak is linked to the theme of prophecy; the woodpecker is a prophetic bird, while the oak is the tree of sacral kingship. How much of this symbolism would have been apparent to Geoffrey's audience is impossible to ascertain, but perhaps less than the more overtly stated Celtic legendary motifs such as the healing fountains or the journey to the Fortunate Island.[3]

CHAPTER 14

I *The Poisoned Apples*
II *The prophecy of Ganieda*

Oh no, True Thomas, she said,
That fruit may not be touched by thee,
For all the plagues that are in Hell
Light on the fruit of this country.

> *Thomas the Rhymer* (Scottish ballad).

Root and branch shall change places, and the newness of the
thing shall pass as a miracle.

> *The Prophecies of Merlin.*

The third Marvellous Appearance is that of a madman (closely
associated with the vision of a strange tree over a fountain). He
is one of Merlin's old comrades, driven mad by poisoned apples
set for Merlin by a frustrated lover. But this madman is finally
cured by that same fountain that cured Merlin, and he joins the
prophet, Ganieda, and Taliesin in spiritual seclusion in the
woods and the astrological Observatory built for them.

Ganieda sees a light shining in the windows of the Observatory,
and falls into a prophetic trance in which she recounts some
events connected to the period of Geoffrey and his readers or
listeners. Merlin finally declares that the mantle of power has
passed from him to his sister; the prophetic spirit has left him. He
has grown beyond seership towards a spiritual and transcendent
consciousness in which such powers are no longer necessary.

THE POISONED APPLES

After he had finished speaking a certain madman came to

them, either by accident or led there by fate; he filled the grove and the air with a terrific clamor and like a wild boar he foamed at the mouth and threatened to attack them. They quickly captured him and made him sit down by them that his remarks might move them to laughter and jokes. When the prophet looked at him more attentively he recollected who he was and groaned from the bottom of his heart, saying, 'This is not the way he used to look when we were in the bloom of our youth, for at that time he was a fair, strong knight and one distinguished by his nobility and his royal race. Him and many others I had with me in the days of my wealth, and I was thought fortunate in having so many good companions, and I was. It happened one time while we were hunting in the lofty mountains of Arwystli that we came to an oak which rose in the air with its broad branches. A fountain flowed there, surrounded on all sides by green grass, whose waters were suitable for human consumption; we were all thirsty and we sat down by it and drank greedily of its pure waters. Then we saw some fragrant apples lying on the tender grass of the familiar bank of the fountain. The man who saw them first quickly gathered them up and gave them to me, laughing at the unexpected gift. I distributed to my companions the apples he had given to me, and I went without any because the pile was not big enough. The others to whom the apples had been given laughed and called me generous, and eagerly attacked and devoured them and complained because there were so few of them.

Without any delay a miserable madness seized this man and all the others; they quickly lost their reason and like dogs bit and tore each other, and foamed at the mouth and rolled about on the ground in a demented state. Finally, they went away like wolves filling the vacant air with howlings. These apples I thought were intended for me and not for them, and later I found out that they were. At that time there was in that district a woman who had formerly been infatuated with me, and had satisfied her love for me during many years. After I had spurned her and had refused to cohabit with her she was suddenly seized with an evil desire to do me harm, and when with all her plotting she could not find any other means of approach, she placed the gifts smeared with poison by the fountain to which I was going to return, planning by this device to injure me if I should chance to find the apples on the grass and eat them. But my good fortune kept me from them, as I have just said. I pray you, make this man drink of the healthful waters of this new fountain so that, if by chance he get back his health, he may know himself and may, while his life lasts, labor with me in these glades in service to God.' This, therefore, the leaders did, and the man who had come there raging drank the water, recovered, and, cured at once recognized his friends.

THE POISONED APPLES

The tale of the poisoned apples gives us the last link in the scrambled and diffused sequence of magical or transformative symbols that relate to Merlin, the power of prophecy, its relationship to insanity or imbalance, and the patterns of polarity.

The madman who appears is one of Merlin's old comrades, and the location at which he was driven mad is described in detail; it is an imaginative location, an inner vision linked to both myth and the natural environment.

In the mountains a great oak tree rises over a spring or fountain; the same area or location in which Merlin first met the messenger with his lyre. It is a primal vision, the world-tree over the fountain of life. In modern mystical texts or magical instruction this tree has been linked to the Qabalistic Tree of Life, but native vegetative tree symbols long predate the arrival of the mathematical Eastern variant.

Lying upon the fragrant grass are apples, ripe and ready to eat; but the fruit of magical places is not all that it might outwardly seem to be. Merlin's companions eagerly gather up this fruit and eat it, and they immediately lose their reason, foam at the mouth, and behave like wild dogs or wolves. This reminds us that Merlin's own companion during his madness was a wolf, and the connection is plain to make. We are encountering a reworking of the madness theme, with a different origin to the imbalance and wildness; the battle and grief motif has been set aside for another and more ancient theme.

Men are driven mad by these apples, which are the poisonous gifts of a woman. This might seem initially to be linked to the Garden of Eden story from the Old Testament, but we should also look to a traditional ballad that deals in detail with the UnderWorld, prophecy, a tree bearing fruit, and the power of a female figure.

In *Thomas the Rhymer* a man is carried off by the Fairy Queen, who rides with him through rivers of water and blood or a roaring sea and red blood, which flow underground. They arrive at a tree, and Thomas offers to pick the fruit for the Queen. She advises him this fruit is tainted with 'all the plagues of hell' and that it must not be eaten by mortal man. It is, in fact, the raw fruit or power of the mysterious UnderWorld, growing upon the Tree of Life. The Queen then offers Thomas bread and wine (the fruit transformed) and carries him to Elfland, where in time he becomes a seer, and eventually returns to the outer or upper world.[1]

The parallels between this ballad, based upon a historical person, and the elements of the Merlin story are striking. Both involve a seer, rivers that flow underground, a tree with potent or poisonous fruit, and a female power of transformation. Both also include a final return to the human world.

Geoffrey is recounting a traditional song or tale which is clearly part of the broad prophetic and magical tradition in which Merlin plays the leading or master-role. The poisoned apples are rationalised to a certain extent, but they are linked correctly with the powers of sexual or procreative polarity: 'after I had refused to cohabit with her . . . she placed the gifts smeared with poison.'

This mysterious woman is likely to be the third aspect of

the feminine triplicity mentioned earlier; she is a dangerous and sometimes violent power. If Ganieda represents the powers of sisterhood and enabling wisdom, and Guendoloena the powers of flowery sensuality, then the Apple-woman represents those fearsome powers of madness and death which were known in the ancient Celtic goddesses. She does not appear as a crone, but her negative power of taking is clear.

It hardly needs to be added that this catalytic force is not wantonly destructive; we have followed Merlin's own career from the wild-man wolf-fervour to that of the wise ancient. Without the prophetic ferment he could not have grown in this manner.

In short, the goddess is a goddess of highly charged inspiration, linked to the sexual energies of the human organism. These energies, which are quite clearly expressed in the *Thomas Rhymer* ballads by the relationship between Thomas and the Queen of Elfland, are transformed or transmuted by the higher consciousness . . . indeed they *are* the source of the higher consciousness. Used in one way they lead to madness and poison, used in another they lead to prophetic vision and mystical realisation. The entire Merlin narrative leads us through this sequence.

Both Thomas and Merlin are characters in a diffused but enduring tradition of changing mystical and magical con-sciousness; we cannot assert that one is derived from the other, even though Thomas is of a later date.[2] They are the leading symbols, based upon historical persons, of a process native to the western psyche; as such we would expect their tales to have a deeper origin than mere literature or entertainment.

THE PROPHECY OF GANIEDA

Then Merlin said, 'You must now go on in the service of God who restored you as you now see yourself, you who for so many years lived in the desert like a wild beast, going

about without a sense of shame. Now that you have
recovered your reason, do not shun the bushes or the green
glades which you inhabited while you were mad, but stay
with me that you may strive to make up in service to God for
the days that the force of madness took from you. From now
on all things shall be in common between you and me in this
service so long as either lives.' At this Maeldinus (for that
was the man's name) said, 'Reverend father, I do not refuse
to do this, for I shall joyfully stay in the woods with you, and
shall worship God with my whole mind, while that spirit, for
which I shall render thanks to your ministry, governs my
trembling limbs.' 'And I shall make a third with you, and
shall despise the things of the world,' said Taliesin. 'I have
spent enough time living in vain, and now is the time to
restore me to myself under your leadership. But you, lords,
go away and defend your cities; it is not fitting that you
should disturb beyond measure our quiet with your talk. You
have applauded my friend enough.'

The chiefs went away, and the three remained, with
Ganieda, the prophet's sister, making a fourth, she who at
length had assumed and was leading a seemly life after the
death of the king who so recently had ruled so many people
by the laws he administered. Now with her brother there was
nothing more pleasant to her than the woods. She too was at
times elevated by the spirit so that she often prophesied to
her friends concerning the future of the kingdom. Thus on a
certain day when she stood in her brother's hall and saw the
windows of the house shining with the sun she uttered these
doubtful words from her doubtful breast.

'I see the city of Oxford filled with helmed men, and the
holy men and the holy bishops bound in fetters by the advice
of the Council, and men shall admire the shepherd's tower
reared on high, and he shall be forced to open it to no
purpose and to his own injury. I see Lincoln walled in by
savage soldiery and two men shut up in it, one of whom
escapes to return with a savage tribe and their chief to the
walls to conquer the cruel soldiers after capturing their
leader. O what a shame it is that the stars should capture the

sun, under whom they sink down, compelled neither by force nor by war! I see two moons in the air near Winchester and two lions acting with too great ferocity, and one man looking at two and another at the same number, and preparing for battle and standing opposed. The others rise up and attack the fourth and savagely but not one of them prevails, for he stands firm and moves his shield and fights back with his weapons and as victor straightway defeats his triple enemy. Two of them he drives across the frozen regions of the north while he gives to the third the mercy that he asks, so that the stars flee through all portions of the fields. The Boar of Brittany, protected by an aged oak, takes away the moon, brandishing swords behind her back. I see two stars engaging in combat with wild beasts beneath the hill of Urien where the people of Gwent and those of Deira met in the reign of the great Coel. O with what sweat the men drip and with what blood the ground while wounds are being given to the foreigners. One star collides with the other and falls into the shadow, hiding its light from the renewed light. Alas what dire famine shall come, so that the north shall inflame her vitals and empty them of the strength of her people. It begins with the Welsh and goes through the chief parts of the kingdom, and forces the wretched people to cross the water. The calves accustomed to live on the milk of the Scottish cows that are dying from the pestilence shall flee. Normans depart and cease to bear weapons through our native realm with your cruel soldiery. There is nothing left with which to feed your greed for you have consumed everything that creative nature has produced in her happy fertility. Christ, aid they people! restrain the lions and give to the country quiet peace and the cessation of wars.'

She did not stop with this and her companions wondered at her, and her brother, who soon came to her, spoke approvingly with friendly words in this manner, 'Sister, does the spirit wish you to foretell future things, since he has closed up my mouth and my book? Therefore this task is given to you; rejoice in it, and under my favor devoted to him speak everything.'

I have brought this song to an end. Therefore, ye Britons, give a wreath to Geoffrey of Monmouth. He is indeed yours for once he sang of your battles and those of your chiefs, and he wrote a book called 'The Deeds of the Britons' which are celebrated throughout the world.

THE PROPHECY OF GANIEDA

The closing scene of the *Vita* consists of Merlin, Taliesin, and Maeldinus the ex-madman retiring to the woods to lead a withdrawn spiritual life. They do not, apparently, live on wild berries and spring water as Merlin did during his madness, for they retire to the special compound built by Ganieda for observation of the stars.

There may be some symbolic structure at work in this fourfold relationship: Merlin is the wise old man, representing consciousness matured through long experience; Taliesin is the learned bard, who represents consciousness matured through formal learning or training as in the Mysteries; Maeldinus is the wild fervour of consciousness brought into balance through the grace of a curative miracle. They are in many ways merely aspects of the compound figure of Merlin as presented through Geoffrey's works and through other equivalent traditions in both Britain and Europe. The three men are another variant of the Three Faces of Merlin, madness and fervour in youth, learning and exposition in adulthood, and timeless experience and wisdom in old age.

Ganieda is the British equivalent of Minerva; she enables the transformative action, manipulates situations to gain specific end results, acts as a sister of wisdom and advice, and builds the complex observatory. In Geoffrey's curious ending to the narrative, she becomes a prophetess in a scene which is quite strongly coloured by what was likely to have been direct experience of the prophetic trance, perhaps from a Welsh seer whom Geoffrey encountered. Ganieda stands in the hall, and sees light shining upon the windows (of the Observatory); this inspires her trance.

The prophecies in this case are very contemporary references, in which certain hopes for Geoffrey's immediate future society are expressed. They are not mystical prophecies in any way, but are a good example of political prophecies. The scene is a carefully stage-managed one.[3]

But the passing of the spirit from Merlin to his sister is not merely a matter of political contrivance, it is in keeping with both the ultimate aim of spiritual enlightenment, and the overall vague connection between Ganieda and an enabling goddess figure from an early culture. Merlin has grown beyond his phase of utterances, and reaches that strange end to all spiritual enlightenment, where the powers sought by the unenlightened are passed over and eventually transformed and outgrown. Ganieda takes the mantle of far-sight upon herself, and perhaps this is right, as it may have originated in her earlier aspects as a Celtic goddess who protected and inspired seers, bards, and prophets.

CHAPTER 15
Synthesis:
Merlin, Mabon and the
Riddle of Three, Four, Six

The North of England still retains a living sword-dance tradition, known as *Rapper*. This tradition is shared with a number of European or Mediterranean cultures; the symbolism of the dance-drama is coherent, and suggestive of ancient religious or mystical exposition. A group of men circle a chosen individual while making a sequence of patterns by interweaving flexible blades with a grip or handle at each end. During the development of the dance a variety of figures are generated from the polarities or possibilities of the numerical combinations involving the six blades or the chosen number of dancers. Six is the number found in Northern English rapper dancing, though other numbers are also known.

The ceremony leads to the apparent beheading of a central figure, yet he may also rise again, sometimes standing upon a platform woven from the dancers' swords. When the celebrants weave inwards for the kill, six blades are linked to form a six-pointed star, hexagram, *Knut* or *Knot*. In modern slang the word *Knut* (nut)[1] is still used to denote the head, and Celtic legends and history both affirm the magical significance of the head from a period of ancient and unknown origin, but at least as early as the encounters and conflicts between head-hunting Celts and the Greek and Roman cultures in the fifth century BC.[2] The head was to develop a symbolic complex of harmonious connectives which persisted well into the medieval period with the Grail legends, and to remain in traditional dance-drama into the twentieth century.

Such is the briefest summary of the dance ceremony, which is dealt with at length in various published studies.[3] We have already introduced a harmonic element into the interpretation which is not generally admitted in standard folklore, but which is nevertheless a working proposition; such ceremonies, no matter how they are preserved or regenerated, have clear symbolic links with the most primal and yet sophisticated Mysteries. Here the word Mystery is used in the specific sense of a spiritual, psychological, and training school or selective system of transpersonal education, such as were known in ancient Egypt or Greece. The Mysteries have a public ritualised element which later developed as theatre, and an inner or esoteric content which was always openly displayed but often undiscovered by the participants.

In the modern remnant of the dance ceremony, the display of the six-pointed star is a moment of triumph and applause, a visible culmination of the complexities of the dancers' steps and mutual pattern-making. All interacting elements, the swords, have merged into a *Knot* or *Lock*, the traditional names for this universal pattern of momentary stability and harmony.

Many comments have been made upon the meaning of the Hexagram, in works which range from ritual magical texts in their most banal or superficial literary form, to learned and mystical expositions based upon both detailed research and inner cognition or perception. During the nineteenth century it was wrongly presumed that the Hexagram was either Eastern in origin or of Hebrew orthodox derivation. The simple fact is that the symbol appears widely throughout human culture, and its presence in various forms in European and Celtic lore demands an individual examination.

We shall take as our point of departure the ritual sword dance of the North of England, a dance with a geographical connection to the ancient kingdom of the Brigantes which covered an area including the modern counties of Yorkshire, Westmorland and Cumberland. This merest fragment of connection will lead us to triple, quadruple and sextuple symbolism in British Celtic tradition; it reveals a series of connectives establishing a deep inner motive for the general retention of oral lore and customs well into the twentieth century. There is no implication of conscious preservation or that the geographical coincidence is 'proof' of anything whatsoever, but we have to enter the weaving patterns somewhere, and a living ritual dramatic tradition can hardly be bettered or denied. It must be stressed that the sword dance or rapper dance is perpetuated by ordinary people as a small but important aspect of their lives; it is emphatically not an intellectual or pseudo-artistic revival, although these also exist in abundance.

The sword-weaving dance, and its European and Mediterranean relatives, is an invaluable indication of the endurance of ritual symbolism within the common imagination. Such symbols are not enacted through any fabricated study on the part of the participants, therefore they are not a 'psychodrama', nor are they part of a formally declared religion, even when the ceremonies are linked to the Catholic calendar that absorbs so many pagan events throughout the year.

We may follow the symbolism back in time through various expressions, until we approach but never penetrate a veil of highly energised archetypical relationships. The word 'archetype' is used here not in the modern psychological sense, but to define a set of matrices that stand before some original source of creative power. The *shape* of these matrices will harmonically determine all subsequent expressive forms; not rigidly but fluidly or musically. The source of the creative power may be either Divine or human, but when we consider ancient traditions this source is mediated through an ancestral or collective pool of experience encapsulated and transmitted in specific sets of symbols.[4] Thus our definition or metaphyscial use of the word 'archetype' is nearer to the classical than the modern meaning, for there are archetypes of universal creation that link harmonically to images of collective imagination. One such enduring symbol, representing an archetype that is both Macrocosmic and Microcosmic, is the Triangle and its doubled or mirrored form, the Hexagram.

In Celtic tradition triple symbolism abounds in numerous, often seemingly disparate expressions. Archaeology, literature, iconography and tradition from oral sources all provide evidence of significant triplicity; triple goddesses, triple hooded figures; triple form in poetry; and triple themes in which relationships between personae are specifically highlighted to form the foundation for all subsequent action, be it tragic, comic or magically irrational.[5]

This triple symbolism is expressed ultimately by the motif known as the Threefold Death, found in many Celtic tales, and deriving from magical or religious practices common to many early cultures. A close connection between the Threefold Death and Christian trinitarian and sacrifical symbolism has often been commented upon, and is not necessary to this brief discussion. Before we draw such great religious parallels, we must first grasp the roots of triple symbolism in our native lore where it long predated the arrival of Christianity and, in a most attenuated form of tales and dances, has survived the decline of orthodox Christian state religion. Such early cultural material does not presume precedence over religion or faith of any formal type; both are harmonically related, deriving from human consciousness wrestling with the mysteries of life. In this sense dogmatic historical or superficially logical lines of relationship are fruitless.

Just as the Knot displayed in traditional sword dancing is a brief expression of an eternal truth, or at least a clear demonstration of disparate units linked in harmony of shape, polarity out of fluidity, so is the display of triple symbolism a momentary locking of other units which are usually thought to be unconnected. Unification, weaving into a six-pointed star, is not merely the product of our intellect seeking to justify itself by finding meaning; the moment of display and applause in the dance, the coherence of exposition in a book or essay, are each aspects of a Mystery revealed. The original matrix is our triple or sextuple pattern; the interplay of subsequent energies represented by the dancers is a result of our varying modes of consciousness. If we can for a moment perceive such energies afresh in their own state or world rather than through derivatives or reactions, we experience them as revelation: the six pointed star.

In ritual drama, a death and resurrection ceremony, a dance of swords, offers its moment of triumph as a hexagon; the dancers have gone through many tortuous, even painful movements to achieve this curious epiphany. In the diffuse realms of early tales and verses, the movements are no less complicated; they have many branches of expression that remain uncrystallised, unpurified by the catalysis of perpetual dance. Nevertheless the archetypes, the matrices, are alive within our root imaginative literature drawn from an oral and profoundly subtle wisdom tradition. The origins of this wisdom tradition will never be found, for it is organic, and schools or religions such as Druidism, Greek or Roman Mysteries, or Christianity, all drew nourishment from those deep strong roots reaching far into the UnderWorld.

To demonstrate the application of triple, quadruple and sextuple symbolism in wisdom tales, we can briefly examine two major sources: *The Mabinogion*, a set of Welsh tales deriving from oral traditions written out during but predating the late medieval period; and the *Vita Merlini*, setting out a collection of earlier poems and traditions relating to Merlin the British prophet. Each of these collections had a profound effect upon literature of later centuries; both act as mediating matrices for concepts emerging from a protean oral source (the common imagination and poetic archive of tradition) into a more rigid written format.

The *Mabinogi*, as they should be called, derive from the lost adventures of the Celtic god-child Mabon.[6] Within the lengthy and racy tales remaining, it is the interchange of polarity, or role between characters that is paramount. A relationship between kingship, sexual interplay, a goddess of the land, and the power of the Other or UnderWorld connects the various tales. Detailed examination of these harmonic themes reveals a pattern of triplicity, with personae merging into one another in a magical manner. In early interpretations, under the convenient rationalisations of 'nature worship' or 'solar mythology', the cycle suggested in the *Mabinogi* was vaguely linked to the

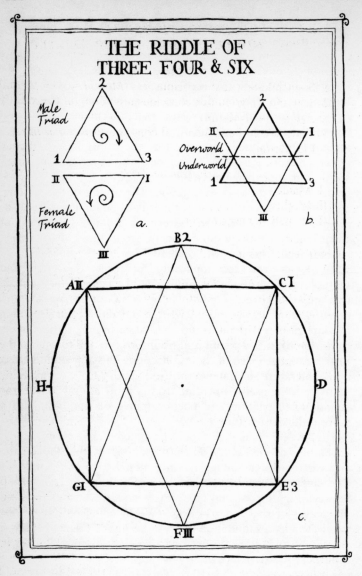

Figure 13 *The Riddle of Three, Four and Six*

KEY TO FIGURE 13:
THE RIDDLE OF THREE, FOUR AND SIX

a Male Triad

1 Son/Child/Spiritual consciousness (*Mabon, young Merlin*)
2 Seer and King/Human consciousness (*Dragon Chief, Arthur, mad Merlin*)
3 UnderWorld Lord/Ancestral consciousness (*Guardians, old Merlin*)

b Female Triad

   I Maiden
  II Mother
 III Shape-Changer or Crone

Both Seer-King (2) and Crone (III) are Shape-Changers

c Triads and Square upon Wheel of Life

A Merlin/Mother (Seer and Goddess)
B Shape-Changer (archetype of Seer-King) Maeldinus, Bladud: EAST
C Guendoloena/Maiden (Flower Maiden, Virgin)
D New Husband (originally god of procreation): SOUTH
E King Rhydderch/UnderWorld Guardian
F Shape-Changer/Crone (archetype of priestess) Morgen, Apple Woman: WEST
G Ganieda/Child (Sister/Foster Mother) Briggida, enabling goddess
H Lady of Stars/Taliesin (Bard of Wisdom and Goddess: NORTH
Centre: *Blessed Youth of Three Changes*

Note: This Figure is a synthesis of the personae and roles found in both the *Mabonogi* and the *Vita Merlini*. To trace its development follow through Figures 2, 4, and 6. For detailed analysis of the personae in the *Mabinogion* refer to Caitlín Matthews, *Mabon and the Mysteries of Britain* (Routledge & Kegan Paul, forthcoming).

Four Seasons; but as we shall see shortly seasonal symbolism is a later stage of the fluid expression of archetypes at their work. The fundamental pattern is threefold. Within a detailed study of the Mystery aspects of the *Mabinogi*, Caitlin Matthews[7] has clarified a triple relationship between male characters, a relationship that spills over into other tales, poems, and legendary themes derived from Celtic lore throughout Europe, and which has further 'Indo-European' parallels and psychological implications worldwide.

The basic roles or characters appear in various guises and under numerous names, but each fulfils a definable function. This definition by function runs through the mythology of the ancient world, and acted as a cohesive inter-cultural psychic or magical force which is sometimes difficult for the modern mind to grasp; while tribes and races were openly ethnocentric in their regional practices, there was a unifying symbolic flow that may have been truly international.[8] Within the *Mabinogi* and similar tales, the male triplicity appears as follows:

1 *Mabon* son of *Modron* ('son, son of Mother'), the Child.
2 Various mature males: *Head* or Chief of the UnderWorld (Pen Annwm).
3 *Arthur*, *Taliesin* and others: *King* or *Bard*. As we shall see shortly, this is a dual function, that of King/Seer, or King/Prophet.

These three merge into one another and react in a cycle reaching through three worlds:

1 The Child (Spiritual or Primal world)
2 The King/Seer (Human and Magical world)
3 The UnderWorld Lord (Ancestral or regenerative world).

(Thus far I have followed Caitlín Matthews' interpretation of roles in the *Mabinogi* fairly closely, but from this point on the analysis is my own.)

The King/Seer manifests in the human world either as a tribal ruler or a giver of poetic and prophetic insight; the divine Child may grow into either role, *according to the need of his people*.

The Triad of roles rotates (Figure 13a) in such a manner that the King/Seer descends into the UnderWorld to liberate his successor, the Child of Light, who in turn becomes the mediator of the new consciousness as King or Seer to the people and the land. The triple cycle is found in many myths worldwide and is by no means confined to Celtic symbolism. It represents great cycles reaching through immense periods of historical time, yet it also epitomises specific reactions or interchanges within the human spirit or psyche.

The Child is our primal source of spirit; the King/Seer is our personality or entity in the outer world; the UnderWorld Lord or Head is ancestral consciousness below and fundamental to our presumed 'selfhood'.

A complete human being has full experience of all three, and such self-knowledge is the avowed and recognised aim of ancient Mysteries. The *Mabinogi* are therefore a genuine expression of the Mysteries of Britain.

The male Triad is the direct sexual counterpart of that female triplicity made known anew in the twentieth century by the late Robert Graves. Graves' highly personal interpretation of the Goddess has sometimes obscured her traditional identity; in his influential book *The White Goddess*, Graves' personal poetic need for a complete system has steered modern literature towards a firm definition of the Goddess in three aspects:

  I Maiden;
 II Mother;
III Crone.

Such a primal Triad is indeed represented in early tales, poems or sagas, and is suggested by some archaeological evidence. The third aspect, however (as Graves clearly states but subsequent writers have lazily oversimplified), is really that of a Shape-Changer. She is that Third Person of a Female Trinity who may be whatever she wills. This may seem to the reader to be a rather trivial example of symbolic thread-picking, but we shall return to this role of shape-changing shortly, being aware initially that transformation is central to human wisdom traditions of all kinds worldwide.

The Female Triad corresponds ideally to the Male Triad as shown in our Figure 13. The relationship is one of polarity rather than mutual identity, thus they are not polar opposites as in stereotypes of male-female relationship, but relate in a more subtle manner. Additionally, the relationships are in a constant state of rotation or flux, but the ideal correspondences are as follows:

Mother/Child (II/1)
Shape Changer/King-Seer (III/2)
Maiden/UnderWorld Lord (I/3)

As the Male Triad rotates through a cycle sunwise (from left to right) so does the Female Triad rotate starwise (from right to left). If we superimpose the Triads upon one another, we have the Hexagram, that same six pointed star displayed in ritual dance from collective and enduring folk tradition (Figure 13b).

The relationships suggested above are not idle speculations; they are embodied in numerous tales, ballads, poems and legends. A mother-child relationship is perhaps the most obvious, but all three require a short elucidation in our present context.

King and Shape-Changer The King represents the fertile or energising effect of people upon the land, or the human race upon the planet. Such beliefs were central to Celtic lore, with kings married in the magical or spiritual sense to the Goddess of the Land. In later Irish tradition, perpetuated in songs and poems well into the nineteenth century, this female spirit of sovereignty still appeared as a mysterious woman who spoke with the voice of the land, expressing popular dreams or almost mystical political hopes. The superficially rational emblem of Brittania devised in England is merely an expression of the figure of sovereignty, or the goddess Brigidda/Minerva, so beloved of the early British people.[9]

We repeatedly find tales in which a king or knight is 'married' to a foul ugly woman who transforms herself into a fair maiden upon the correct answers being given to certain riddles or trick questions.[10] The land, or the planet, is *protean*, but it is polarised or rendered fair (or in the present times foul) by marriage to human consciousness. More simply we could also say that male and female energies within the psyche must be in a balanced marriage to one another; but this type of valid rationalisation sidesteps the issues clearly defined by early symbolic marriages, in which the connection between humans and the environment is explicitly stated.

UnderWorld Lord/Maiden A virgin or maid is mythically linked to the powers under the earth; the chief or head of that potent realm, the UnderWorld, is her Guardian. A hero-king may not liberate her alone, he requires the aid of a company of specifically gifted heroes, and finally must seek the aid of the Child of Light, a spiritual power permeating the worlds. In this manner the triple cycle of the male Triad, described above, is rotated. We may note that the stimulus is the connection between virginity (in the sense of both sexual and spiritual grace) and the guarding or protecting power of the Under-World, from which all energies and secrets are revealed or concealed. The passage of the Maiden from the Giant or Guardian to her intended mate the King is not merely a matter of sexual fertility, but harmonically connects to both individual and cultural development, maturity, even civilisation.[11]

Mother and Child The Maiden becomes the Mother after her union with the King, and a mysterious Child is born to initiate a new cycle. The Child, however, in the *Mabinogi*, is hidden or stolen away.

As the Male and Female Triads rotate the number of relationships is not limited to those primary connections defined above; the flow of polarities is always fluid, with the triadic map providing a key to the potential links between male and female, be they people or archetypical matrices for creative power. It is the function of the Mysteries to lock the archetypes together for a timeless time, fusing them in such a manner that they resonate through into the human psyche or outer world . . . and so the dancers display their six-point star of swords.

It should be stressed at this stage in the argument that keys such as the diagrams and analyses described are not a substitute for the real thing; the myths, legends and related wisdom lore from collective tradition must be experienced directly. There is no value whatsoever in applying the systems outlined above and below in a merely intellectual or superficially enquiring correlating manner; the connections will be found, the patterns revealed within characters or mythic themes, and long (tedious) lists of correspondences may be drawn up. All of this is trivia and dross without a living reaction from within ourselves. Originally the patterns which we are discussing were applied directly in daily life, at a time when life and ritual magic were hardly separate.

Mere superstition plays little part in such ritual weaving, and the connectives are deep rather than coincidental. As each layer of the fabric is carefully drawn aside, a further pattern is revealed, until we begin to approach that which is concealed below: the origins of consciousness, be it that of a man, a woman, a tribe, a planet, or a star.

We move now from the polarity analysis of the *Mabinogi* to that of the *Vita Merlini*, our second working example. This text restates a cycle of magical and ultimately spiritual development epitomised through the figure of Merlin. Many of the traditional or widespread elements incorporated by Geoffrey of Monmouth share themes found in the *Mabinogi* which were almost undoubtedly current in a number of forms in Wales at the time in which Geoffrey was writing. Material is also drawn into the *Vita* from post-classical encyclopedic sources, exempla, and Geoffrey's own earlier monumental work *The History of the British Kings*, which incorporates *The Prophecies of Merlin*.[12]

The *Vita* contains cosmology, magical geography, natural history, and a guided tour of the Celtic Otherworld. The plot, which is a masterful exposition of curative psychology, gives us Merlin growing through a series of transformations (psychic rather than physical); he progresses from his first appearance as a mad frenzied seer-king to becoming a fully enlightened and spiritually liberated elder who has a memory extending through long periods of time. In this progression he is following the triadic theme found in the *Mabinogi* and other traditional sources: Seer-king to ancient Guardian. In *The Prophecies*,

Geoffrey's earlier collection of Merlinic lore, Merlin utters the future history of Britain while still a youth, with a curious parentage of virgin wed to otherworld being.

Thus Merlin exhibits the presumed *Mabon* cycle of divine youth, adventures through time, imprisonment, liberation, great age beyond that of mortal span, and other attributes which are closely worked into the narrative. Unlike the *Mabinogi*, the *Vita* holds fast to a compassionate psychology or spiritual resolution dealing with individual problems. Merlin poses the questions asked by all humans: about death, hardship, grief, love, the future, worldly and spiritual values and so forth. But his questions are answered in remarkable depth, each being turned from a human complaint into a revelation of the Mysteries, for Merlin is undergoing the path of initiation.

Just as primal polarities are revealed by the *Mabinogi*, so are seasonal and sexual polarities dealt with in the *Vita*, overlaying the primal triads but never totally obscuring them. It is in the *Vita* that we may find seasonal, human, and transpersonal cycles integrated with the triadic primal (Titanic) cycles of earlier lore. The briefest summary of patterns found in the *Vita* is shown in our Figure 6. The spiritual growth of Merlin is enabled by interaction within a square of sexual or sibling relationships, set upon the circle of the four seasons. Each major persona stands at the corner corresponding to his or her seasonal attributes or elemental nature. In this sense alone, the *Vita* is one of the earliest maps of psychological types, but it uses this definition of personae or personalities as one part of a vast harmonic conceptual system.

The four major characters form two sets of pairs, sexual partners and brother/sister interactions:

1 Merlin and his wife Guendoloena; Winter and Spring.
2 King Rhydderch and his wife Ganieda; Summer and Autumn.

Ganieda is the sister of Merlin, while Guendoloena is a type of flower-maiden, the sensual 'sister' of Rhydderch who is a king of summer, the worldly powers. We shall see shortly that those roles overlay primal figures found in myth and legend.[13]

Merlin travels around a spiral of the seasons; his journey is beset by hardship, but enabled by his sister Ganieda, who may be partly identified with the goddess Minerva (the Roman form of Brigidda or Brigit).

The personal role of the characters who square the circle, which means that they stand for us all upon the Wheel of Life, is echoed and supported by four further characters, each redolent of magical and spiritual power from a culture which long predates that of Geoffrey's medieval/Celtic biography. These four are only vaguely defined, but their functions are clear enough for us to grasp that they are the origins of which the personae are reflections (although most literary commentators see them as reflections or poetic conceits based upon the major personae). One of these four, the bard Taliesin, plays a bridging or mediating role for elucidated wisdom, and curiously he also acts as a bridge between the two sets of characters, between the personae and the archetypes, having the nature of both.[14]

1 Maeldinus: a wild frenzied man of the woods, inflamed by the juice of poisoned (i.e. magical) apples.

2 The New Husband: a male figure who replaces Merlin in the sensual affections of Guendoloena when she is rejected in favour of a life of prophetic or spiritual withdrawal. His only function is to appear in a tower window and be ritually slain by Merlin.

3 The Apple Woman: an ex-lover of Merlin, who seeks to poison him with apples set out beneath a great tree. She actually poisons (inflames with prophetic madness) Maeldinus, revealing the connection between the goddess and the seer or madman.

4 Taliesin, a bard of wisdom, who is specifically stated as being under the instruction of Minerva.[15]

These four stand behind or beyond the Quarters of the Wheel; they are rationalisations or controlled expressions of the mythic and religious figures found worldwide. We might summarise them as follows:

1 EAST: The Lord of the Animals; Wild Spirit; the Lord of
   the Swarms.
2 SOUTH: The Lord of Generation; male power.
3 WEST: The Lady of Sacred Fruit; Queen of Elfland; Lady
   of the Worlds or Spheres.
4 NORTH: The Lady of Wisdom; Lady of the Stars. She
   speaks through Taliesin who reveals the mysteries of the
   Universe to Merlin, and defines the bridge between the
   Macrocosm and Microcosm during a lengthy dissertation
   on stars, planets, powers, daemons, and natural life upon
   the planet Earth. We find this stellar lore running
   continually through the Merlin texts, in which a type of
   observational astrology is combined with prophetic vision,
   seasonal astronomy with inspiration.

In the *Vita*, therefore, Geoffrey has included those traditional
roles also found in the *Mabinogi* and other wisdom tales. King,
Seer, Maiden or Mother are well defined, and the UnderWorld
Lord appears as the persona of Rhydderch, in the guise of a
worldly king. But his function is clear: he enchains and even
tempts the prophet, who is not freed until questions are
answered. It is the death of Rhydderch which finally frees
Ganieda (Rhydderch's wife and Merlin's sister) to join her
brother in a specially constructed spiritual-stellar observatory.
In this final scene, Ganieda is accompanied by Merlin,
Maeldinus, and Taliesin: a male triad join asexually to a female
central figure.

The primal roles are mixed in the *Vita*, but as we have stated
earlier the triads revolve and are not necessarily in the ideal
configuration demanded by literary analysis. This configuration,
like the star of swords, is a symbol of revelation rather than of
logic, but like all revelations it may be reduced to a series of
logically related images, stories, motifs, songs and dances.

There are a number of other characters in the *Vita Merlini*
who are directly pertinent to our theme, and as is often the case
with such mythical/magical/pagan religious personae, they are
found in many guises in many tales throughout British or Celtic
lore. The simplest way to deal with these characters in brief is

to list their attributes rather than their numerous cross-references:[16]

1 *King Bladud*: a shape-changing flying priest-king who
   guards sacred springs and wells and is especially connected
   to the Temple of Minerva at Aquae Sulis, Bath, England.
   Bladud ('Light-Dark') acts as Janus or entry warden for
   Merlin, Taliesin and the wounded King Arthur to sail to
   the mysterious Otherworld. With his consort queen *Aleron*
   (possibly meaning 'wings' from the French 'aileron')
   Bladud plays an important role in the mystical cosmology
   revealed to Merlin by Taliesin in the *Vita*. Bladud is, in
   fact, the archetype of the King/Seer, the male shape-
   changer.

2 *Barinthus*: a supernatural ferryman who knows the seas
   and stars, and steers the magical vessel holding Arthur and
   the two companions to the Fortunate Island.

3 *Morgen*: rules the Island; she is also a shape-changing
   flying person, derived from a traditional goddess image.
   She has Nine Sisters (three times three) and is the
   innerworld counterpart of the male shape-changer. Just as
   Bladud marks the entry to the sacred wells and springs, so
   does Morgen rule over the island reached by sailing on the
   mysterious UnderWorld or Otherworld sea. Like Bladud,
   Morgen is also concerned with healing, and promises to
   cure Arthur, but only after a long time in her keeping. The
   implications of Arthur's failure to keep the kingdom whole
   are discussed elsewhere.[17]

The role of seer-king is one of shape-changing, and this is by
no means a rationalisation of primitive ceremony which
modern writers identify all too easily with 'shamanism'. Such
kings undergo totem beast transformation, flight, future-vision,
rapid changes of size and strength; they may also be rulers of
great power and wisdom, or may be sacrificed *in time* for the
benefit of their people, land, or planet. Just as it was convenient
to label such themes as 'solar myths' during the last century, it
is nowadays convenient to label them as 'shamanism'. Neither
label truly describes the theme and neither approaches a

genuine understanding of the many harmonic levels involved ... of which solar myth and shamanistic practice are
but two of the more superficial or obvious.

The triadic patterns underpin a holistic structure in which
human, environment, planet, and stellar patterns are inseparably and musically related. The matter of time is central to this
holism, for the rotations may manifest as a real historical
person over a short time-scale, or as a great and cosmic change
of order over a stellar time-scale. Whatever the apparently
relative time involved, the cycles are perpetual. But certain
individuals, and Merlin was one, are able to break free first of
the tiny human cycle, and then to work their way through the
entire related cycle of cycles; this is clearly represented by
Merlin as a youth who nevertheless had a vision that reached to
the very end of the solar system: the end of planetary time as
far as humans are concerned.[18] This liberation theme is central
to Celtic legend, for it is the liberation of the *Mabon* or Child
of Light, shown in the ritual sword dance by the elevation of
the central figure upon his starry platform, but also by another
shape which we shall meet with shortly.

The feminine role of curative transformative goddess is also
one of shape-changing. She is the inner or Otherworld
counterpart of the seer-king who lives in the human world. In
Celtic seership the power of prophecy always derives from this
goddess or feminine power of consciousness; in Celtic kingship
the royal right to rule is derived from a union with the feminine
power of the Land.

Shared motifs, common to both the *Mabinogi* and the *Vita*,
include the marriage of a Flower Maiden,[19] the power and age
of certain totem beasts,[20] an overbearing kingly or Titanic
power,[21] the duty and role of both kingship and seership,[22] the
journey to the UnderWorld,[23] and the curative nature of
spiritual enlightenment.[24] In the sword dance the man who is
ritually slain, apparently decapitated, is a harmonic of that
mysterious Head of Bran, central to one of the major themes of
the *Mabinogi*.[25] In some examples from genuine folk tradition,
the ritual dance is included in a drama (Mummer's Play) in
which a role-changing man-woman and a quack doctor preside

over the death and resurrection of a hero or of a child. And this in the nineteenth and twentieth centuries of industry, reason, materialism, waste, plastic, and nuclear incurable pollution!

It remains to us now to ask who is that central character, killed, resurrected, elevated? As we are not dealing with religious parallels, we shall not go any further into the death, ressurection, and divine ascent of Christ. In Celtic lore, which is essentially pre-Christian lore, we can identify this person as the victim of the Threefold Death. In the *Vita*, the *Mabinogi* and a series of related tales, someone undergoes a strange multiple death, often in a ritualised and highly symbolic set of circumstances. In the *Mabinogi*, it is *Lleu* who is ritually wounded while in a most bizarre pose that is reminiscent of the imagery of a Mystery or of a god. *Lleu* is a not too distant relative of *Lugh*, the ancient god of Light. In the Scottish tales of *Lailoken* which are close to the narrative employed by Geoffrey in the *Vita Merlini*, it is the prophet himself ('Lailoken who some call Merlin') who is impaled, stoned, and drowned, after predicting this triple death to a Christian saint.[26]

The *Vita*, however, offers us a curious and significant variation, one which is often passed over by literary commentators as being a mere contrivance to draw the sacrificial death away from Merlin so that Geoffrey might keep his central character to the very end of the poem. A youth appears in a dramatic scene engineered by Ganieda to disprove Merlin's powers of far-sight.[27] Firstly he comes as himself with long hair, secondly with his hair cut, and thirdly dressed as a girl. The importance of hair-cutting and the coming of age of a hero are found in the *Mabinogi*,[28] while the sexual role assumption is reminiscent of the ritual dramas (Mummers Plays) referred to above.[29] One central youth changes role or shape, and so represents all men and women. Perhaps Geoffrey's variant is a true representation of a Mystery enactment. The youth dies all three deaths predicted by Merlin: falling from a height while hunting, hanging by one foot from a tree, and so drowning in the river below.

This image is almost identical with the Tarot Trump of the *Hanged Man*, in which a beatific individual hangs from a curious tree by one foot. Tarot cards, however, were not formalised until at least three centuries after Geoffrey wrote and assembled his *Vita*.[30]

The Threefold Death is a variant, a primal expression, of the theme of the Sacrificed Innocent God found in religion worldwide. Thus we have: a triple male cycle, a triple female cycle, triple role-playing by a youth, and a triple death. The four-square sexual seasonal and elemental powers are centralised by the youth (the *Mabon*) and his Threefold Death: falling to Earth, hanging from the Tree of Life, drowning in the depths of the UnderWorld waters.

As we are told by both religious and mystical teachings, and by the cycles of nature herself, this Threefold Death is the prelude to a return to life.

We may, therefore, find the Youth at the centre of the Wheel of Life as squared by the personae of the *Vita Merlini* (Figure 6) and at the centre of the Hexagram formed by the primal Triads suggested in the *Mabinogi*. As a Youth he is neither Child, King-Seer nor UnderWorld Lord, neither Mother, Maiden, nor Crone; in short, he is neither male nor female but partakes of both equally, resolving them through a third spiritual transcendent function.

The primal Triads of male-female relationship indicate the traditional theme of the manifestation of spirit into matter (known in orthodox religions as the Fall, and shown as a set of triads upon the Qabalistic Tree of Life). The second set of matrices, that of the Wheel of Life, four seasons, and human relationships attuned to archetypical Otherworld beings, is a working key towards the restoration of matter through the action of spirit. There is no implication of sin, guilt, damnation, or punishment in these sequences, as they predate Christian political propaganda.

The various elements of the *Vita* are synthesised in our Figure 4 and the relationship between the polarity square and the primal Triads is shown in Figure 13b.

The *Mabon* cycle reveals primal powers in triadic relationship, while the *Merlin* cycle (mainly in the *Vita* but including *The Prophecies* and their setting in *The History of The British*

Kings) reveals how such powers transform and ultimately mature the psyche in our growth towards spiritual enlightenment.

At the ending of the dance, after the decapitation, the resurrection, the elevation upon a six-pointed star . . . what then? Does the victim merely return to the weaving patterns to be killed and reborn again and again? Not so, for after the display of the Hexagram and our applause, the swords are unwoven, the Wheel dissolved, the Universe unmade. Such cosmic lore is found in *The Prophecies*[31] more than in the *Vita*, but there is one important visual key hidden but displayed openly in Geoffrey's mystical psychology, just as it is hidden and displayed in the folk dance from the region of the Brigantes, children of the goddess Brigidda.

In the dance, the company performs a curious stepping over the swords, almost a contortion performed by sleight of hand. It seems that they take an impossible step that will tie them up in knots or tangles, for it goes contrary to common sense or to the circular motion of the dance itself, the round of the seasons, the Wheel of Life. But they take this step, and emerge from it freely; it is the secret step shown by the Threefold Death, by the Hanged Man.

Although there is no implication here that traditional dancers have any intellectually conscious plan or 'secret knowledge' regarding their symbolism, which is perpetuated from generation to generation by the enduring strength of the shape, the dance, the tradition itself rather than any commentary or interpretation, such mystical and magical steps were definitely known to the early Church. In the case of the Church the knowledge was conscious, though soon to be suppressed, for it was drawn directly from the pagan Mysteries through the membership of early Fathers in Mystery cults prior to their conversion. Furthermore, such wisdom did not merely evaporate with the advent of the Roman state Church, but endured in forms which gradually became absorbed through the oral primal traditions rather than intentional initiations or ceremonies. To take our discussion into its last phase, we should hear from Saint Thomas Aquinas:

Now in the movement of bodies [i.e. entities of any type] the more perfect and primary ones have position. Therefore the principal spiritual operations are described under this appearance as three different movements: *circular* whereby anything is moved uniformly around its centre; *straight* whereby a thing proceeds directly from one point to another; the third is *serpentine* which is made up of both circular and straight.[32]

This passage from Aquinas reiterates an ancient metaphysical teaching which appears also upon the Qabalistic Tree of Life. Within the seemingly straight line, across the apparently closed circle, flows an element of unpredictable motion. This is the power sought in the higher working of ritual magic; in mysticism and religion it corresponds to the 'Spirit that bloweth where it listeth'. It also lives within each of us. When this power is activated or brought through from its own world or dimension into any other, it cuts across all regular lines, modes or cycles of operation, and is not bound by the regular sets of laws that govern manifest creation. Traditionally the straight line is equated with God the Father; the circle with the Virgin or the Mother; the serpentine motion with the Son of Light, who is the product of their active union. This primal or gnostic Christian type of exposition was later replaced by the orthodox trinity of Father, Son and Holy Ghost. The Ghost or Spirit, however, was originally the first point or breath of origin, the seed in the centre of the circle.

We find this conceptual model, resonating closely to those of the *Mabinogi* and the *Merlin* poems, in an anonymous thirteenth-century song *Cum Sint Difficilia*:

Cum sint difficilia Salomoni tria
quartum nescit penitus quod est viri via
in adolescentula quod est Christi transitus
in Virgine Maria.

(Solomon has difficulty with threes, the fourth he plainly does not know, which is the way of man into a young girl, which is the passing of Christ into the Virgin Mary.)

> Hec est adolescentula que soli Verbo patula
> quod fuit ab initio. Sic patet quod non partitur
> cum intrat aut egreditur,
> quia Verbi conceptio sine contagio
> partus sine vestigio.

(She is a young girl who alone was receptive of the Word which is from the beginning. Clearly she feels nothing when the Word enters or passes from her, because the conception of the Word is free of contagion and the birth without vestige.)

> Ipsa nihilominus terra coelum mare.
> ipse quoniam Dominus serpens avis est et navis
> cuius non difficile sed impossibile vias investigare.

(She is nevertheless the Earth, the Sky, the Sea. He, as he is Lord, is a Serpent, a Bird, and a Ship whose ways are not difficult but impossible to investigate.)

The origin of this curious devotional song is French, but it retains symbolic features which could easily be Celtic in origin, just as many of the poems and romances of the same culture retained equally Celtic motifs fused with Christian esoteric lore. The song demands a study in its own right which cannot be undertaken here, but like the triadic power-matrices described above, it offers a triple female and triple male pattern merged in sexual, but not merely sensual, unity. The Serpent in the Earth, the Bird in the Sky, and the Ship on the Sea all play major symbolic roles in both the *Mabinogi* and the *Vita Merlini*. It is also worth observing that the word-play upon 'vestigio' and 'investigare' derives from a most ancient Mystery of Birth, found in the *Mabinogi*, merely hinted at in the birth of Merlin, and reappearing in the symbolism of the Order of the Garter.[33]

The Threefold Death of the *Vita Merlini* and other multiple deaths encountered in myth and legend are inevitably connected to an unusual assembly or fusion of the four Elements: Air, Fire, Water, and Earth. The overall concept expressed is that a rotation or combination of the Elements leads to a magical and spiritually attuned 'death'. This theme is well represented in alchemical emblems and texts which inherited the vast store of symbolic wisdom cast aside by the orthodox Churches. On a divine religious level the pattern is that of the Crucifixion and the attendant death, descent into Hell, and final spiritual elevation of Jesus. Within the individual it manifests as a powerful transformation of the psychic-body complexity, the total entity that comprises a human being. This is the traditional 'living death' of the initiate into the Mysteries, a transformation in which a spiritual rebirth is undertaken while still alive within the physical or consensual world, rather than after physical death.

In a short summary of this sort there is not space to catalogue and compare the various types of multiple death found in tradition, or to closely analyse the links to Christian symbolism. We will, instead, return directly to that Threefold Death described by Geoffrey in the *Vita Merlini*.[34]

A youth appears in three roles or guises, then dies a triple death by *falling, hanging*, and *drowning*. This death combines the Four Elements as follows: falling from a great height = Air; hanging upside down from a tree = Fire to Earth, crossing the Abyss from light to darkness by the most direct path; drowning = Water. If we locate this triple death or triple movement upon the Wheel of Life, it travels East, South, North, West. This *serpentine* motion cuts across the Wheel, and acts as a path of liberation from the cycles of life, death, and rebirth (see Figure 12). The crossed legs of the Tarot image of the Hanged Man suggest this secret path, and he is a figure of spiritual peace, not of material suffering.

In Eastern traditions such as Tibetan Bhuddism, the secret path is that taken by the seed-syllable Aum resonating through the physical and metaphysical worlds. In Christianity it is the path taken by Christ to enter into the human world, an esoteric theme which played an important role in Gnostic teaching, and still features today in Qabalistic mysticism. In Celtic lore, as we have seen, it is the path of the Threefold Death by which the Seer-King invokes the Son of Light, suspends the Triadic cycles, and declares Peace. Operations of this type are well defined by meditational, religious, and magical practices worldwide;

whatever form they take, whatever tradition they follow, they reveal a deep and important response from human conscious-ness to its *location* within a world of worlds.

Most significant of all in our present context, the Path is that of the lightning flash of liberation; it is the serpentine way taken by the *Mabon* (Child of Spirit) as he is freed from his UnderWorld chains and dances West, North, South, East.

These ancient mysteries of *direction* remain vital to the physical transformations that follow upon metaphysical trans-formations; they manifest in ourselves as the result of our inner disciplines or efforts, they manifest in the physical universe as the result of immense energetic interplays of polarity still mysterious to our advanced physics, and they manifest symbolically in the patterns of traditional ritual dance. So our investigation, in the company of Merlin, of the mysteries of Three, Four, and Six, begins and ends with the Child who Dances.

> But as for me, if thou wouldst know what I was;
> In a word I am the Word who did dance all things
> and was not shamed at all.
> 'Twas I who leapt and danced.
> But do thou understand all, and understanding say:
> Glory thee, Father . . . Amen.

(And having danced these things with us, beloved, the Lord went forth. And we, as though beside ourselves or wakened out of deep sleep, fled each our several ways.)[35]

CHAPTER 16
Conclusions

1 The *Vita Merlini* is a synthesis of exemplary tales and mystical/cosmological teaching.

2 Although the units of the *Vita* (the differing sub-poems and educational sections) come from a wide number of sources both classical, post-classical and Celtic, they show a subtle interrelationship.

3 The interrelationship is energised through the personal hardships, transformations, and psychic-sexual interactions of Merlin. There are repeated indications of an older sub-stratum of magical, mystical or pagan religious narrative which also holds the assembled material together, again through attributes and adventures of Merlin and his immediate relatives or associates.

4 Many of the Celtic mythical themes are found in parallel wisdom tales which reveal elements of the *Vita* to be part of a general myth: the story of the First and Last Man. Aspects of this are found in Merlin's relationship to the Seasons, to animals, to other men and women, and to his final understanding of the links between the Microcosm or human world and the Macrocosm or superhuman world. In this respect, seasonal questions, the Wheel of Life, are related harmonically to stellar questions, the Wheel of the Heavens.

5 Differing from related tales of Celtic seers, the *Vita Merlini* deliberately contains a spiritual resolution, in which the prophetic powers are outgrown and spiritual contemplation becomes the aim of life. The *Vita* contains, therefore, an *active* harmonisation between Celtic pagan lore and Christian faith, rather than a passive change in which the pagan seer is merely 'forgiven' before his death.

6 Many if not all of the above elements have clear value and
   practical application to modern mystical, meditational,
   magical and spiritual disciplines.

II

The length and detailed exposition of many parts of the
narrative are likely to be difficult or even tedious to the modern
reader, and there is a temptation to see these as mere padding or
copying on the part of the author/assembler, Geoffrey of
Monmouth. But the long educational sections are not merely
quotations from reference sources, they have various harmonic
changes, additions, subtractions, and are very carefully placed
with respect to Merlin's transformations and growth towards
spiritual enlightenment. To understand these sections, we must
consider them in cultural context; not only did the medieval
author apply to learned sources continually with reassuring
repetition for support to his arguments, but such passages in
the *Vita* echo an older pattern. The epic narrative is central to
cultures with an oral tradition of entertainment and wisdom;
Geoffrey's Norman-British audience would have had some
contact with a culture or sub-culture in which the epic narrative
was a regular occurrence. Long involved tales and recitations,
have been known in the Hebrides as late as the twentieth
century, so persistent was the story-telling tradition in Celtic
areas.

During the twelfth century, the Welsh and Bretons had a vast
store of poems, songs, narratives and recitations, many
fragments of which are preserved in collections, which include
of course Geoffrey's own work among many others. It is likely
that Geoffrey was quite deliberately reworking the native epic
narrative/wisdom cycle into a stylish Latin with classical
learned allusions for his sophisticated (or relatively sophisticated) audience.

7 The *Vita* acts as an interface between a fragmented oral
   epic cycle of initiation, magical transformation, and

psychic development and (a) literary developments in subsequent texts, (b) classical myths and legends which also include similar transpersonal themes. The classical allusions are likely to be the additions of Geoffrey first and foremost, though we have no way of knowing if his source or sources within bardic traditions also drew classical Greek and Roman parallels by the twelfth century. It seems very likely that they did so, if we judge the evidence of other Welsh fragments or poems in which a wide range of learning is exhibited.

8 There is a practical element to the *Vita* which is best demonstrated by a summary of the Images and People (given in appendices I and II). The dynamics of the text may be applied in visualisation or meditation, as they are the dynamics of the human psyche and its interactions.

9 The *Vita* displays a clear proto-psychology centuries before modern materialist theories were first provocatively voiced in the late nineteenth century. Allowing that its technical terminology is different, and that it relies mainly on imagery rather than intellectual assembly, the *Vita* is a most perceptive handbook of the human psyche and its resultant behaviour. This level of the *Vita* is valid even if one rejects the deeper mystical and spiritual teachings which were the avowed purpose of the author/assembler.

10 Many of the specific elements of the text are coming back into the general imagination and consciousness in the late twentieth century; the powerfully independent woman who is the equal of any man; the rejection of sexual stereotypes; the dubious value of materialism; the growth of transpersonal or paranormal powers within the individual; the seeking of a harmonic or universal worldview that is not merely a dogmatic religious statement or a materialist behaviouralist reduction to absurdity; the emphasis on the feminine principles of consciousness within the human psyche; the assertion that a relationship with Nature as a holistic cycle or life-form is essential to human health and development: these

are all central propositions of the *Vita Merlini*.

11 Although the *Vita* is a British or European book, it holds
those universal or transcendent truths that are evident in
many of the great religious texts worldwide; it is a
neglected but major spiritual text in its own right.

12 The Life of Merlin is an exemplary magical and spiritual
life-pattern for the transpersonal growth of the Western
psyche; it demonstrates clearly the feminine and
masculine powers and polarities in a systematic
development leading to a continuing insight. At its
conclusion, Merlin does not die (as in related tales) or
become seduced by a maiden (as in later moralistic
rationalisations), but travels on to the unending
contemplation of the divine being. Furthermore, his
completeness is a shared unity, for a balanced entity is
fused together by the characters of Merlin, Ganieda,
Taliesin, and Maeldinus. They form a group in which
personal desires, sexual stereotypes and worldly values
have not been rejected (as they have all experienced the
cycles of such activities) but have been outgrown.
Poetically we might say that from their Observatory, they
move into a new dimension among the stars, in which the
heavens and earth are unified through a balanced
humankind.

There can be no greater aim for us today than that which
was achieved by the Mystic Life of Merlin.

APPENDIX I
Images

Each image is described in the order in which it appears in the narrative of the *Vita*. Certain images recur, and many are typical magical, meditative, or religious images. Though they are rationalised in the text of the *Vita*, these images reveal a wealth of information and harmonic connections when they are considered as pictures or visions. The original poems or songs about Merlin and the *Vita* itself would have been declaimed or read to a mainly illiterate audience. The atmosphere of this type of entertainment, as anyone who has heard traditional ballads or sagas will affirm, is one in which images are perpetually generated in the collective imagination of the audience. The same images also form the foundation-stones of the collective consciousness of the culture.

1   Merlin as mature man, a ruler over his people.
2   Merlin watching a terrible battle.
3   Merlin as Wild Man in the woods, with a wolf as companion.
4   Merlin sitting by a fountain on a mountaintop . . . nuts fall from the trees around him.
4a A messenger plays a lyre to the prophet seated by the fountain.
5   Merlin meets two women: one lush and bright, the other thoughtful and dark. They emerge from a thorny pathway to greet him.
6   Merlin with messenger standing before the throne of King Rhydderch, who is an archetypical ruler.
7   Merlin chained to a stake or to a tree stump.
8   Merlin standing before the King and Queen, while a youth appears in Three Disguises.

189

9   Image of the Threefold Death, in which a man hangs by
     his foot from a tree with his head in a river. He has died
     by breaking his neck, falling from a height, and
     drowning.

10   Merlin raging to escape out of the city gates, with two
     women to his right and left, trying to stop him.

11   Merlin upon a hilltop watching the stars at night. One
     bright star emits two clear rays.

12   Merlin riding upon a stag and leading a herd of wild
     animals.

12a Merlin throws horns into a tall tower window, killing
     a man who leans out.

12b Merlin falls off the back of a stag into a flowing river,
     pursued by a troop of men.

13   Merlin again bound at the court of the King (as 7 above).

14   Merlin being taken forcibly through a market-place
     crowded with people. (Confronts a beggar, and a brash
     youth.)

15   Merlin debating with his sister at the city gates.

16   The Observatory built in a remote place; it has seventy
     doors, seventy windows, and an order of attendant
     scribes. It is supervised by Ganieda. (A sub-image might
     be the actual building of the site, with the labourers and
     the Queen directing their task.)

17   Taliesin and Merlin relate the Creation of the Worlds.
     Two men standing before a cosmic vision imprinted in
     the sky, showing the various circles of the heavens, stars,
     planets, clouds, seas.

18   Merlin, Taliesin and Arthur in a boat by night. They are
     steered by the mysterious figure of Barinthus, who
     follows the stars to keep course.

19   Arthur upon a golden bed, attended by Morgen,
     surrounded by her Nine Sisters.

12   Merlin as an extremely ancient man. This is the third
     aspect of the Three Faces of Merlin (youth, maturity,
     old age).

13   Merlin at the Healing Fountain, dipping his head into
     the flowing water.

14   Merlin watching a flight of cranes making mysterious
     letters in the sky. This is a parallel image to that of
     Merlin watching the stars; both are concerned with a
     mystical alphabet that transcends regular cognition, but
     is harmonically attuned to Nature.

14a Merlin watching a woodpecker in the ancient oak tree.

15   The Poisoned Apples: a giant oak tree rising over a
     fountain, with apples lying upon the grass at its foot.
     Several people are running amok or frothing at the
     mouth, but a young Merlin stands looking on. Close to
     the tree is the partially hidden figure of woman.

16   Merlin curing a mad wild-man, by taking him to the
     Healing Fountain.

17   Merlin, Taliesin, Maeldinus and Ganieda together. The
     wise old man/the learned bard/the wild man/the
     enabling feminine spirit. The Observatory (perhaps a
     stone circle) is in the background.

18   Ganieda looking upon a bright light in the window of
     the Observatory. (This is reminiscent of the goddess
     Minerva and her perpetual light that burnt at the temple
     of Aquae Sulis; of Saint Brigit and the perpetual flame
     that burnt in the monastery of Kildare.)

These are not the only images available within the *Vita*, but are
those which stand out as magical or visionary images of key
significance. Any one of these could, for example, be used in
meditation as a subject for creative imagination.

SIMILARITIES BETWEEN IMAGES IN
MERLIN TEXTS AND TAROT TRUMPS

Both *The Prophecies* and the *Vita* clearly state images which
are in many ways identical or close to the later development of
the Tarot trumps in Renaissance theosophy and magical
symbolism. As the major images have been dealt with at length
either in the preceding chapters or in *The Prophetic Vision of
Merlin*, a short summary only is included here.

Merlin image	Tarot trump
1 Stellar/Solar/Lunar exposition and general imagery of the cosmos (*Vita*). General images of Signs relate here (*The Prophecies*).	STAR/SUN/MOON
2 Taliesin (*Vita*): the master of the Mysteries.	HIEROPHANT
3 Merlin as old man in spiritual retreat (*Vita*).	THE HERMIT
4 Goddess raising dust of Ancients (*The Prophecies*).	JUDGEMENT
5 The Threefold Death (*Vita*).	HANGED MAN
6 Apocalyptic Vision (*The Prophecies*). Passing of Rhydderch (*Vita*). (The first is on a cosmic level, the second a human level.)	DEATH
7 King Rhydderch (*Vita*).	EMPEROR
8 Symbolism of sign of Libra (*The Prophecies*). The trial of Merlin's vision linked to the Threefold Death motif (*Vita*). The Judge of the dead beneath the Earth (*Vita*), harmonically linked to 4 above.	JUSTICE
9 Vortigern's ruined Tower (*The Prophecies*). The Tower of the usurping lover (*Vita*).	BLASTED TOWER
10 Figure wrestling with lion (*The Prophecies*).	STRENGTH
11 Malign star shown as Saturn or Orion (*The Prophecies*).	THE DEVIL

Merlin as wild man wearing horns or
connected to horned animals (*Vita*).

12	Merlin and Guendoloena (*Vita*).	THE LOVERS
13	Ganieda (*Vita*). Figures of maidens or goddesses found in various aspects (*The Prophecies*).	THE EMPRESS
14	Morgen (*Vita*). Figures of various maidens etc. (*The Prophecies*). The images of 13 and 14 may be inter-changeable to a certain extent, depending upon the function of the female figure in its specific place in the narrative of either text.	THE PRIESTESS
15	Imagery of cyclical changes (*The Prophecies*). Imagery of Merlin's cycle of change (*Vita*). Fourfold imagery of both *The Prophecies and Vita*. Image of Ariadne's Wheel (implied in *The Prophecies*).	WHEEL OF FORTUNE
16	Merlin as young man (*The Prophecies*) Messenger image (*Vita*).	MAGICIAN
17	Creation of the World (*Vita*). Goddess of the Land (*The Prophecies*).	THE WORLD
18	Merlin with wolf in woods (*Vita*). Young man pursuing hounds to his death, and youth in varying disguises (both in *Vita*).	THE FOOL
19	The Charioteer of York (*The Prophecies*).	THE CHARIOT

The Tarot image of *Temperance* is not correlated.

It must be stressed that these connections are not merely the intellectual or superficial result of juggling with the images. To gain the best critical understanding, the reader should examine each of the Tarot trumps mentioned (either in the traditional pack or the A.E. Waite design based upon Renaissance cards) and compare it with the vivid images in the Merlin texts. A further set of corresponding images is found in the minor cards drawn for the Waite Tarot pack, but these are not valid for listing in the present context, as they were produced in the early twentieth century, whereas the trumps are genuine images from the early Renaissance period. There can be little doubt from an unprejudiced examination of the Merlin images and the later Tarot trumps that they have many connections, both in image and in meaning.

The list given is not definitive; there are a number of further connections that the reader can find by examining the texts. The *Vita* is more suited for establishing clear images than *The Prophecies* due to the protean and chaotic nature of much of the imagery in the previsions of Merlin, but both texts hold the foundations of a cycle of images which were later restated in the Tarot trumps.

APPENDIX II
People

There are several major characters in the *Vita Merlini*; interaction between them is vital to the development of the narrative, and to Merlin's own maturity through experience, insight, and education.

The relationships between characters are generally overt and defined (husband and wife, brother and sister) but certain apparently minor people play significant roles that demand closer examination. Mythical persons also appear in minor but important roles.

MAJOR CHARACTERS: Merlin; Ganieda; Guendoloena; Rhydderch; Taliesin.
MINOR CHARACTERS: A Messenger; A Youth; Maeldinus (a madman); a Woman (spurned by Merlin); King Arthur.
MYTHICAL CHARACTERS: Bladud (a British god-king); Minerva (a goddess); Barinthus (a supernatural guide or ferryman); Morgen (a goddess); King Arthur.

Arthur is cited as both mythological and as a minor character, as his role in the *Vita* is primarily as a mythic figure in the legend of the wounded king and the Fortunate Isle.

The short lists above represent the people who have key roles in the sub-text and main narrative, and who act as essential factors in the mythical, magical, psychological and spiritual relationships and symbols of the text. They are dealt with in our main analysis of each section of the narrative, but a summary of each person may be helpful in defining their function. Each individual figure is described with regard to his or her magical or psychological role, and not in the context of historical or literary sources which have been amply dealt with in other studies.

MAJOR CHARACTERS

Merlin

The major prophet of the Western esoteric traditions. He has three primary aspects: young man inspired by inner visions, mature man tormented by strife and guilt or compassion, old wise man who endures beyond all human experience.

Merlin has a number of clear parallels to Jesus, and may be derived from a pagan tradition similar to that which was transformed by the Christian incarnation, death, and resurrection.

Merlin	Jesus
Born of a maiden and a spirit.	Born of a Virgin and the Holy Spirit.
Makes oracular announcements.	Makes oracular announcements.
King Vortigern tries to sacrifice Merlin as a youth.	King Herod massacres the Innocents.
Merlin's mother is of a royal house.	The Virgin is of royal lineage.
Merlin confronts false magicians and confounds them as a youth.	Jesus confronts elders in the Temple as a youth.
Retires to wildwood through madness, grief or compassion leading to prophecy.	Retires to desert to meditate.

Is tempted by King Rhydderch with the gifts of the world.	Is tempted by Satan with rulership of the world.
Is associated with an ancient theme of ritual sacrifice (the Threefold Death).	Is crucified.

At this stage, the close parallels end, as the Christian resurrection is of a different order to the life of Merlin. Merlin represents an ancient pagan method of insight and inner growth, while Jesus represents similar themes but upon a higher level. Other significant parallel symbols are: Merlin associated with UnderWorld energies/Jesus descends to Hell to liberate souls; Merlin rejects the normal sexual pattern of relationship/-Jesus rejects the normal sexual pattern of relationship; Merlin associated with miraculous cures/Jesus performs miraculous cures; Merlin berates worldly powers (in *The Prophecies*)/Jesus berates worldly aspirations.

There is no implication that Merlin was contrived as a false imitation of Christ, but that the major themes of both are drawn from an enduring tradition with recognisable elements that relate to human inner or spiritual growth.

Merlin acts in both *The Prophecies* and the *Vita* as the epitome of the Western prophetic consciousness in action. He teaches through example and through symbols of insight, rather than through direct or intellectual exposition. Towards the close of his life, Merlin grows beyond prophetic powers and retires to the woods for spiritual contemplation.

The older elements of Merlin are connected to a primal seasonal myth in which a wild man of the woods, ruler of animals, relates to a flower maiden who represents the fertile earth. The seasonal cycle is partly reflected in the progress of Merlin during the narrative development of the *Vita*.

Merlin also commands certain cosmic or transcendent powers of vision; these are the ultimate end of prophecy rather than mere far-sight or prediction. In this role he is intimately connected to a female divinity, who appears as either a guiding or enabling figure (Minerva) or a weaving power who both assembles and unravels the solar system (Ariadne).

In literary analyses of Merlin two figures are assumed to have been conflated by Geoffrey of Monmouth: Merlin Ambrosius, founded upon an earlier Merddyn figure in Welsh tradition, and Merlin Calidonius, based upon a tradition known in Scotland. The first encompasses *The Prophecies* while the second brings in the wild-man theme of the *Vita*. Both 'Merlins', however, share a great deal; they are impelled to their insight through matters of strife or polar relationships (fighting dragons or fighting armies or personal conflict within the consciousness). It is more likely that both figures represent branches of a common oral tradition which retained the wisdom songs or poems of the old Celtic/Druidic culture, preserved in bardic entertainments such as those confirmed by various chroniclers. This central issue of transformation through polarised energies is dealt with fully in our analyses of *The Prophecies* and of the *Vita*.

Merlin, therefore, symbolises the core tradition of Western psychology, magic, and mysticism. This tradition involves inner transformation and growth through radical changes in modes of consciousness which are linked to the archetypical figure of a goddess. During stages of transition, the prophetic powers manifest in a variety of ways, but are eventually outgrown.

Ganieda

The sister of Merlin, and wife of King Rhydderch. Her function in the *Vita* is complex and essential to the development of the plot.

Ganieda is an *enabling* power; she sends out messengers to bring Merlin back from the wild; she challenges him to deal with the problem of his abandoned wife; she builds his Observatory to gather star-lore; she finally joins him in spiritual withdrawal after the death of her husband.

It is Ganieda who arranges the curious ritualised scene in which the ancient Threefold Death image is brought into the narrative, and she is responsible for most of the controlled action and progress during Merlin's contact with civilisation. There are some significant connections between the figure of Ganieda and that of Minerva. Both arrange the inner and outer progress of a hero or male character who undertakes mythic tasks. Both are concerned with the civilising influences of cultural development upon wild or untamed consciousness; both are 'sister' figures rather than 'lover' figures; both are aspects of a multiple female figure which represents the phases of a goddess in appearance. In the *Vita* Ganieda is connected to Guendoloena, Merlin's wife, who is the epitome of the sexual female, while a third mysterious woman brings madness through poisoned fruit towards the close of the narrative. These three are faint echoes of an ancient triple goddess, representing three aspects of feminine consciousness and three cosmic powers.

Guendoloena

Merlin's wife, image of a sensual or sexual woman. On this first level she is left behind by Merlin during his prophetic madness and his initial wild retreat from civilisation. Later she is the subject of a reasoned rejection brought about through Ganieda's concern for her future; the wife of a hermit, initiate, or wild man is similar to a widow.

Guendoloena is not merely a stereotype, nor is she a lesser character than Ganieda, although she disappears from the story without further explanation. She is the image of a goddess of nature, fashioned out of flowers, a being of intense fertility and beauty. She cannot, in fact, exist alone as a stereotype, for she is complemented and fulfilled by her male partner. Merlin as a wild man is likewise fulfilled by Guendoloena, and the *Vita* barely hides an ancient theme in which the two lovers play the seasonal roles of Winter and Spring, Lord of the Animals and Lady of the Flowers, Death and Life.

The combination of Guendoloena and Ganieda, lover and sister, is perhaps more than a human link through their sharing of love for Merlin. They represent aspects of a goddess, each reacting in her own way to the consciousness represented by the prophet. When Merlin kills Guendoloena's new husband by hurling stag-horns at him, this may be an echo of an ancient ritual struggle between two male images striving for the love of a goddess; but it also equally represents an important truth: the sensual or sexual energies are at the mercy of the wild driving energies of nature, they cannot exist as stereotypical ends in their own right. Once the mock-male has been slain by the wild man, the sensual flower woman merely vanishes away; the potent energies are being used in a new direction which ultimately leads to Merlin's spiritual enlightenment and cure.

King Rhydderch

Husband of Ganieda, Merlin's sister. The perfect worldly ruler, vested with every good quality. He represents to a certain extent those worldly or outward-looking values that the mystic leaves behind; in this role he acts as the tempter of Merlin, offering him rich gifts to remain at court. He is married to Ganieda, but is clearly subservient to her, as the motif of her unfaithfulness is not pursued and is merely a prelude to the scene of the Threefold Death prophecy. The material, outward-looking world-view is ultimately ruled by a deeper, further-reaching consciousness; if necessary this feminine principle of consciousness will betray the regular patterns of the psyche or its world-view in order to demonstrate deeper insights.

Like Guendoloena, Merlin's wife, Rhydderch leaves the story after a new level of inner growth has been reached by Merlin. Upon Rhydderch's death a lament is uttered; he is still a model to the worldly man, his passing away is a model of our mortal doom.

Taliesin

A bard and instructor in the Mysteries of the cosmos. The original Taliesin was a magical child in Welsh legend, and many poems, riddles and traditional fragments of lore are ascribed to him. In the context of the *Vita*, however, Taliesin is primarily a man of profound learning; he represents wisdom through instruction. His teachings are not merely intellectual, but a combination of mysticism, vision, and the 'bardic science' of the classical and Celtic cultures, in which natural phenomena were seen as manifestations of supernatural archetypical forces through a harmonic or holistic series of interactions. This world-view is now beginning to command new attention as materialist science falls into disrepute.

Taliesin answers Merlin's key questions, questions which are asked and answered on several different levels throughout the narrative. It is Taliesin who provides an overview that enables Merlin (and the reader or listener) to rise above purely seasonal or personal difficulties and observe them as part of a master-model in which the universe, the solar system, the planet, and the mysterious Otherworld or UnderWorld are linked together.

Taliesin joins Merlin in his final retreat; instruction and reasoned mystical symbolism join with great experience and wisdom. It is also Taliesin who accompanies Arthur and Merlin to the mysterious Otherworld where Morgen will cure the wounded king.

MINOR CHARACTERS

The Messenger

The Messenger plays the *crwth* or lyre to cure Merlin's fits of madness. He is a symbol of Hermes, the questing intellect, sent by Ganieda (in her role as Minerva), the protectress of heroes and builder of culture. The Messenger is found in a number of other traditional songs, tales, and legends, and always has a magical power or sanctity attached due to his derivation from a god-form known throughout the ancient world. The Messenger is linked to the power of music, which in early cultures was planetary in its symbolic use. It is after the arrival of the Messenger that Merlin's mad prophetic fits become rationalised into planetary symbolism. The Messenger is one of the 'minor' characters in the *Vita* who plays an extremely important pivotal symbolic role in the growth of Merlin towards mystical insight and spiritual maturity.

The Youth

An archetypical dramatic figure. He is the victim of a sacrificial rite in which the victim is hung from a tree, drowned, and has his neck broken. Other variants of this Threefold death use slightly different methods. The youth also appears in a curious motif in which he wears three disguises, similar to those found in traditional dramas or folk ceremonies worldwide. This drama precedes the sacrificial death. He is a symbol of every man and woman; in esoteric terms he is both the repeated incarnation of souls in different guises, and the core mystery of the spiritual sacrifice which was epitomised by the figure of Jesus. The Youth is also a variant of Merlin himself, for in other narratives, the seer predicts the Threefold Death for himself, and eventually suffers it.

Maeldinus

A madman, who represents the state of Merlin's own madness in a reflection theme that occurs towards the close of the *Vita* once Merlin has been cured. He has eaten of poisoned apples, a magical theme found in several variants. Maeldinus finally retires to the woods with Merlin, Ganieda, and Taliesin, making a triple 'Merlin' team of three men and a 'goddess' in the form of the enabling sister. Maeldinus is the power of wildness, madness, and inner ferment of rising energy which can occur if the psyche is overloaded by mystical or metaphysical experience. By his cure at the miraculous spring and his joining with the other characters, he becomes whole. Although a 'minor' character, he reminds us that each aspect of Merlin (Merlin's Three Faces) must be merged and unified to make a balanced psyche or spiritual being.

The Apple Woman

Spurned by Merlin, she is the mistress of poisoned apples. This very vague figure is the remnant of a goddess or Fairy Queen who controls the potent fruits of the UnderWorld, which bless or curse according to the recipient's state of grace. She completes the suggestive trio of women who play such a powerful part in the overall adventures of Merlin; she is the death-woman. While not overtly stated, her role is unmistakable.

MYTHICAL CHARACTERS

King Bladud

First mentioned in *The History*, King Bladud is an important British mythological figure. His attributes are: flying through the air; practising necromancy; worshipping Minerva; patron of healing springs (at Bath). He is also linked with the figure of Appollo, and represents a combined solar deity and the basic functions of the Celtic king and priest. His name is likely to be derived from BEL and DYDD, meaning Light-Dark. His dual nature links him also to the classical figure of Janus, who is mentioned in *The Prophecies* as the doorkeeper of the goddess Ariadne at the ending of the solar system. In the *Vita* Bladud appears during the cosmological teaching of Taliesin, where the springs and wells are encountered before lists of magical islands. In Celtic tradition, the magical Otherworld is often underground or through a well or spring. In other traditions not included in the *Vita* but also of native Welsh or Celtic origin, both Bladud and Merlin have the Pig as their totem animal; a theme which occurs in the legend of the dark goddess Cerridwen whose symbol was the Sow, and in a hunting scene in the Mabinogion where a giant boar is pursued.

Minerva

The classical Roman name that encompasses a number of related goddesses, including the Greek Athena and the Celtic Brigidda. A goddess of light, culture, inventions, education, and patroness of the development of the mind over the passions. Minerva also aids certain heroes upon mythical tasks, including themes in which the Golden Apples of the Hesperides, a tradition associated with Britain, are the object of the quest. She guides Taliesin in his long harmonic exposition upon the Creation of the World, and seems to be the archetype behind the figure of Ganieda, Merlin's sister. Minerva represents the guiding and enabling powers of the feminine principle in the growth of civilisation. Like a number of ancient goddesses, her earliest form is that of a goddess of war, and in this aspect she is connected to similar figures such as the Celtic Morrigan, a triple goddess of fertility, death, and battle.

We may find echoes of this ancient goddess uttered throughout the *Vita*; battle drives Merlin mad, fertility is shown through his wife Guendoloena, death through the mysterious Apple Woman, his spurned lover. The sensible and balanced powers of Minerva are found in the musical cure of Merlin, in the building of his Observatory, in the various decisions and actions taken by Ganieda.

Barinthus

A mythical Ferryman who knows the ways of sea and stars. He carries Arthur, Merlin and Taliesin to the Fortunate Isle. This figure, barely mentioned in the *Vita* as if Geoffrey's listeners might know all about him without further explanation, or as if Geoffrey's oral sources knew the name in some form very well, is another *enabling* image. Barinthus, related to the legendary isles in other Celtic tales, is a power of transportation, not merely in the literal sense, but metaphysically. In a psychological sense he is the archetypical Ferryman who guides us across unknown seas. As a magical or meditational figure, he is a divine guide who guarantees safe passage towards the realms of the Otherworld.

Morgen

With her nine sisters, an Otherworld feminine power, a goddess or Druidess. Her image is likely to be derived from the cult of the native goddess who may be triple or multifold in her aspects. The name reflects a fairly widespread female persona with magical attributes. She flies through the air, changes shape (as does King Bladud) and can cure illness or wounds. She takes charge of the wounded Arthur, declaring that he will have to stay with her on her magical island for a long period of time, but that she will eventually be able to make him whole. This is one of the earliest appearances of the 'wounded king' theme that was to become widespread in Grail literature during the medieval period. Morgen is the regenerative power of the Otherworld.

King Arthur

Arthur appears both as historical king and mythical king in the *Vita*, with his mythical appearance taking precedence and the historical or pseudo-historical account acting as support to the myth. In his wounded state, his passage to the Fortunate Isles with Merlin and Taliesin, his long rest upon a golden bed under the care of Morgen, Arthur is a potent symbol of both the land and the human psyche or spirit. His wound is that disastrous condition arising out of disunity and imbalance (a lesser harmonic of the Fall of Lucifer) which afflicts us all in one way or another. His journey across the sea, guided by Barinthus, is in the company of Merlin (wild prophetic fervour and power) and Taliesin (learned bardic symbolism and education). Arthur, therefore, represents the psyche or spirit carried forth upon the unknown sea of the universe accompanied by the two extreme polarities of its own potential nature. He is a king who has temporarily laid aside his crown and land due to the wounds of battle; a theme reiterated in the *Vita* through the madness and retreat of Merlin.

Arthur is taken in by Morgen, a divine or magical power of regeneration, but the passage of time is spoken of, and repeated by Merlin in his Prophecies concerning the restoration of the Land of Britain. Arthur upon his golden bed in the Fortunate Isle is the origin of those mystical king images found in the Grail legends, or rather all such images devolve from an intuition regarding the condition of the human soul and the symbols of its regeneration.

APPENDIX III
Preiddeu Annwm

THE SPOILS OF ANNWM
(Old Welsh poem)

Praise to the Lord, Supreme Ruler of the Heavens,
Who has extended his dominion to the shore of the world.
Complete was the prison of Gwair in Caer Sidi
Through the spite of Pwyll and Pryderi.
No one before him went into it.
A heavy blue chain firmly held the youth,
And for the spoils of Annwm gloomily he sings
And till doom shall he continue his song.
Thrice the fullness of Prydwen we went into it,
Except seven, none returned from Caer Sidi.

Am I not a candidate for fame, to be heard in song?
In Caer Pedryvan four times revolving,
The first world from the cauldron, when was it spoken?
By the breath of Nine Damsels it is gently warmed.
Is it not the cauldron of the chief of Annwm
Fashioned with a ridge around its edge of pearls?
It will not boil the food of coward or of one foresworn,
A sword bright flashing to him will be brought
And left in the hand of Lleminawg,
And before the portals of the cold place
The horns of light shall be burning.
And when we went with Arthur in his splendid labours
Except seven none returned from Caer Vediwid.

Am I not a candidate for fame to be heard in song?
In the four-cornered enclosure in the island of the strong
*   door,*
Where the twilight and the black of night move together,
Bright wine was the drink of the host.
Three times the fullness of Prydwen we went on sea,
Except seven none returned from Caer Rigor.

I will not allow praise to mere lords of literature;
Beyond Caer Wydr they behold not the prowess of Arthur.
Three times twenty hundred men stood upon the wall,
It was difficult to converse with their sentinel.
Three times the fullness of Prydwen we went with Arthur,
Except seven, none returned from Caer Colur.
I will not allow praise to men with trailing shields,
They know not on what day or who caused it
Or at what hour of the splendid day Cwy was born,
Or who prevented him from going to the dales of Devwy.
They know not the brindled ox with his thick head band
And seven score knobs on his collar.
And when we went with Arthur of mournful memory
Except seven, none returned from Caer Vandwy.

I will not allow praise to men of drooping courage
They know not on what day the chief arose,
Or at what hour of the splendid day the owner was born,
Or what animal they keep of the silver head.
When we went with Arthur of mournful contention,
Except seven, none returned from Caer Ochren.

This curious verse has several parallels with the symbolism employed by Geoffrey in the *Vita Merlini*, particularly in the scene where Arthur is carried to the Fortunate Isle. Shared elements between the *Vita* and the *Preiddeu* include: Imprisonment and chaining motif; use of a ship (Prydwen) to reach a magical realm: fourfold symbolism of the Elements; Nine Maidens; portal symbolism and polarity symbolism (which also feature in the apocalyptic vision of Merlin in *The Prophecies*).

Commentaries upon this poem are found in Graves, R., *The White Goddess*, and Spence, L., *Mysteries of Britain*.

We might add that in the *Spoils of Annwm* Arthur and his host seek to take the magical cauldron of power from the mysterious castle (the various 'Caers') and bring it back to the human world. The portal symbolism and the mixture of night and twilight show that this is the same realm referred to in *The Prophecies* where Janus guards the door of Ariadne, who unweaves the solar system. If this vessel, undoubtedly a type of Grail, had been successfully achieved, it would have brought paradise upon earth. But Arthur's realm failed, and in a later vision, we see the wounded king being returned to the magical place (the Fortunate Isle) for his cure.

It is significant that in another Celtic legend, the cauldron brings dead men back to life (the Mabinogion). Here are the faint echoes of a myth in which the plundering of a sacred vessel leads to chaos and imbalance, a state shown by the ruin of the land and the 'honourable wound' of Arthur. We find it again in a later Grail text in which an order of well-maidens are violated and their cups broken, leading to a ruined land. To rebalance the wasted land, to have his wound cured, we find Arthur (in the *Vita*) being carried to the mysterious Otherworld, where he has to be treated by the goddess herself.

The fact that these themes are scattered through poems and texts spread over several centuries does not in any way affect the harmonic mythical unity that links them; they are connected by images and concepts, as well as by their people. Arthur's failure, therefore, was not in trying to bring into the material world that which belongs in the spiritual world, but in choosing the wrong time, or acting in the wrong manner.

APPENDIX IV
Creation poems

1   TALIESIN'S CREATION POEM
(Extract)

Has not the Skilful One wonderfully covered over Heaven,
   his sanctuary,
With stars and signs and sun and moon?
Daily the sun wheels round the circle of the earth,
On high from above he gives light to
The five zones framed by the all-good Creator.
Sicut in cælo et in terra.
The two furthest of these are full of snow and ice,
And on account of their great cold no one can go near them.
Other two are placed on the under side (of these),
Full of parching heat and burning fires.
The fifth is the middle one, no one inhabits it
On account of the extreme heat of the sun in his course.
The two which come on all sides are of a good temperature;
They receive heat from that side and cold from this.
God erected two fountains of perfect goodness:
A fountain of heat in the air, the sun revolves in it:
And another fountain which produces the waters of the sea.
He created heaven and created everything good,
And created the present state for the children of Adam,
And created Paradise as an abiding place for whoso shall be
   good,
And Hell for the wicked for their destruction.

From the *Myvyrian Archaiology,*
translated by D.W. Nash.

2   GREAT SONG OF THE WORLD

I will adore my Father,
My God, my strengthener,
Who infused through my head,
A Soul to direct me.
Who has made for me in perception,
My seven faculties.
Of fire and earth,
And water and air,
And mist and flowers,
And southerly wind.

And I foresay,
Seven airs there are,
Above the astronomer,
And three parts the seas,
How they strike on all sides.
How great and wonderful,
The world, not of one form,
Did God make above,
On the planets.
He made Sol . . .

And the seventh Saturnus,
The good God made
Five zones of the earth,
For as long as it will last
One is cold,
And the second is cold,
And the third is heat,
Disagreeable, unprofitable.
The fourth, paradise,
The people will contain.
The fifth is the temperate,
And the gates of the universe.
Extract from *The Four Ancient Books of Wales,*
Skene.

APPENDIX V
Lailoken and Suibhne

LAILOKEN (Scottish origin)

A man is driven mad through guilt at causing a great battle and slaughter; his name is Lailoken, though some say it is Merlin. He meets St Kentigern, and eventually asks for the sacrament as his death is impending. Kentigern ascertains the man's Christianity, but is troubled by his habit of prophesying. He tests Lailoken's sanity by asking what the nature of the impending death might be; three questions received three different answers (stoning, impalement, and drowning).

Immediately after receiving the sacrament, Lailoken is killed by the methods predicted. Local tradition in Scotland adds that his triple death at the hands of local shepherds was in vengeance for his giving up the pagan faith, but this is a rationalisation of the tale, albeit one in an unusual direction.

A variant of the tale includes Lailoken predicting the adultery of the wife of King Meldred, and his desire to be buried where the River Tweed and the Powsail burn meet. This was to give rise to Thomas Rhymer's prophecy (thirteenth century):

> When Tweed and Powsail meet at Merlin's grave
> Then England and Scotland shall one monarch have.

Local tradition asserts that the two streams flooded and met together at the ancient standing stone still known as 'Merlin's Grave' when James the Sixth came to the combined throne of Scotland and England.

The parallels with the story of Merlin in Geoffrey's *Vita* are clear. For a full translation of both Lailoken tales see Clarke (Introduction, note 1).

THE FRENZY OF SUIBHNE (Irish origin)

King Suibhne is a pagan ruler who opposes Saint Ronan. Ronan curses Suibhne, who is driven mad during a battle. He wanders around Ireland living on water-cress and spring water, and various attempts are made to capture him. He was eventually given the sacrament by St Moling and died through a spear blow from a jealous husband who suspected him of adultery. Thus was Ronan's curse fulfilled.

APPENDIX VI
The Flower Maiden

They went therefore to Math the son of Mathonwy. 'Well', said Math, 'we will seek, I and thou, by charms and illusion to form a wife for him out of flowers.' So they took the blossoms of the oak, and the blossoms of the broom, and the blossoms of the meadowsweet, and produced from them a maiden, the fairest and most graceful that man ever saw. And they gave her the name of Blodeuwedd, (which means Flower-Face).

Math the Son of Mathonwy; The Mabinogion,
trans. Lady C. Guest.

First she had a great abundance of hair, flowing and curling about her divine neck; on the crown of her head she bore many garlands interlaced with flowers, and in the middle of her forehead was plain circlet in fashion of a mirror born up on either side by serpents that seemed to rise from the furrows of the earth, and above this blades of corn were displayed. Her vestment was of the finest linen of variegated colours, sometimes white and shining, sometimes yellow as the crocus, sometimes rosy red or flaming . . . round about the border of her goodly robe was an unbroken wreath made of all the flowers and fruits.

Apuleius, *Golden Ass,*
extract from description of the goddess Isis.

APPENDIX VII
The Threefold Death and the Elements

The image described in the *Vita* is our Figure 5. It is a specific variant of a widespread magical and spiritual imaginative key, and may be employed in a number of ways.

MEDITATION

1 Using the illustration as a starting point, we build the image in our own consciousness, initially by studying the picture and letting it fill our field of attention. This first stage is sufficient in itself . . . to absorb and be attuned to the image, without intellectual speculation upon its 'meaning'. This is a standard technique of meditation worldwide, and is both the simplest and the most advanced method of using such key images. When the consciousness starts to wander, we redirect our attention to the image; when we begin to speculate upon relationships or meanings, we again return our awareness to the image, holding it in our imagination and visual field, becoming united with it. This exercise is greatly aided by regular repetition.

2 After some practice with the first exercise, we move to building the image solely within our visual consciousness, with eyes closed. In this second phase of the visualisation, we instil the scene with as much life and colour as possible . . . until it becomes a real inner landscape and not a flat image upon a background.

It is at this stage that the image responds to our attention by generating colours, certain intuitive patterns, and perhaps some small but specific changes to its assembly. Any major change, intrusion, or absurdity must be banished by returning to exercise 1. We are not interested, at this stage, in other aspects or characters entering the inner landscape, though these may apply in later developments.

Neither stage 1 or 2 has included speculation on the meaning of the image, but by stage 2 we may begin to pick up intuitive signals from within ourselves, which are the true meaning of such images, of far greater value than any intellectual summary. The intuitive relationship to a meditational image is one of the most important results of this type of work, and will produce known and specific modes of consciousness highly coloured by individual response.

There is no stereotypical or rule-of-thumb effect in the Mysteries, and they are not judged upon spurious merit, grade, degree or intensity of individual responses or abilities. This makes the esoteric lore particularly paradoxical to the modern person who has grown up in a 'meritocracy', for there are no rules or badges to define success; in fact there is no 'success' in the general sense of gaining superiority or material benefit.

The meditation will bring understanding and a sense of right relationship to the symbolism; this works on a level that is not accessible to verbal description, but which is by no means obscure or rare, for it is the imaginative and sometimes dream-like level in which meaning and comprehension are found non-verbally. This state is experienced by us all continually to a greater or lesser degree in waking consciousness and during sleep. In defined visualisation we open it out, and allow it to grow naturally through the defining matrix of the symbol or symbols employed as our starting point. It leads to levels of direct comprehension that may be retranslated into verbal or mathematical units. In science great discoveries are intuited in this manner, while in art the same leap of cognition may be translated into form (image, music, poetry) for sharing with others. In either case, the deeper understanding manifests through serial time as a pattern of 'results'. In the system represented by Merlin, as in all genuine spiritual schools of development, the 'results' are changes within ourselves.

THE SYMBOLISM

It would be unreasonable to exclude some intellectual interpretation of the image of the Threefold Death, although this dissection of the image should not be allowed to disrupt phases of meditation.

The correlations given below are not complete, nor are they rigid or definitive. In general tuition, the student is encouraged to take notes of his or her intuitions after each meditation session, though experienced workers often abandon this discipline. If you are not a practised meditator within Western disciplines (Eastern methods are rather different and may have to be unlearned) the setting out of notes is a valuable experience, and often clarifies many details or intuitions which flee the regular awareness on emergence from meditation, or upon return to customary attitudes and activity.

The Four Elements of the Wise

The image is founded upon the Four Elements of AIR, FIRE, WATER and EARTH. These occur in many places in the *Vita Merlini* as they are the foundations of the classical and medieval world-views. They also comprise the roots of a very ancient and effective metaphysical conceptual model, which we find explained by Merlin and Taliesin in the vision of the Creation of The World (Chapter 10).

We should regard the Elements as elements of Consciousness; in the Creation it is the consciousness of Divinity, while in a general sense the Elements are modes or phases of our own consciousness. These modes are very similar to the physical phenomena defined by the Elements – Air, Fire, Water, and Earth. One of the basic training images of the Mysteries shows a circle divided into four equal parts (see Figure 2) with the harmonic attributes of the Elements in their appropriate places in each Quarter.

Set out in this manner, the Circled Cross is an idealised model; it gives us a theoretical pattern of balance and primal relationship that holds good for both the outer and inner worlds, hence its inclusion in the *Vita* as a universal creation glyph.

Once this wheel is set in motion, many powerful interactions are possible, and the ancient astrological symbolism still employed today is based upon one such system of interactions. In magical imagery, however, we concentrate upon very specific and multifold keys to those interactions which have a catalytic effect upon our consciousness.

Let us consider each of the Four Elements within the image of the Threefold Death (or Hanged Man) and discover how they relate to one another:

AIR The youth falls through the Air to his death; his fall is a kind of flight, reminiscent of the myths in which a male figure attempts to fly to the Sun (Icarus, or in British mythology, King Bladud). His fall is occasioned by various factors: (a) impetuosity, (b) madness or excessive zeal in pursuit of game, (c) ascending to a high mountain. These are typical attributes of the active effects of the mystical element of Air. Air generates certain effects within the psyche: inspiration, excitement, change, energy.

FIRE Is not overtly stated in the *Vita* variant of the Threefold Death, but is implied in a number of ways:
(a) transformation or purification of the sacrificial victim;
(b) his initial hunting frenzy, in which the element of Air ignites his inner Fire (a process also partially outlined by Merlin in his Prayer, where he describes the effects of curative spring water upon his organism (see Chapter 12). The symbol of riding upon a horse is traditionally linked to Fire, as the Horse is representative of great energy and strength in motion; the Tarot trump The Sun shows an innocent child riding upon a great horse, in which the sun is

the central Fire source of our lives. Other Celtic 'death' tales specify Fire in connection with a magical death either through burning or through the use of Fire to heat a magical Cauldron. *Fire* brings incandescence, heat, and illumination.

WATER The victim drowns; related to this is his appearance in disguise as a maiden, for Water is traditionally a feminine element regardless of its appearance in a physically male gender or personality.

The River is the river that washes away past imbalances; it appears as time in the outer world, but as grace in spiritual dimensions. *Time* cleanses through interaction and reincarnation, a concept hinted at by the ritual presentation of the victim in three gender-orientated roles similar to those of life-death-resurrection dramas worldwide. In inner or spiritual states, however, the apparently serial nature of time is found to be an illusion, and it is *grace* or the flow of spiritual understanding (seen by us as blessing or forgiveness) that forms the river.

The victim hangs upside down; his regular world-view has been turned inside out; his head is within the flow of Water. Merlin similarly dips his head into the healing waters that appear by grace at the foot of the mountain (Chapter 12), waters which have been flowing from unseen sources to meet him when they break forth into the serial or consensual outer world as a fountain. The victim's hair spreads out through the flowing river, indicating that his awareness is no longer bound by the superficial limits of his body-identity. Merlin falls from a stag into the river and is captured (Chapter 7), and this may represent an inversion of the image, for he is carried back to the outer world of King Rhydderch's court. The interplay between the encapsulated image of the Threefold Death and elements of Merlin's own career is worth repeating; Merlin's adventures are a cycle or spiral, opening out the central symbolic image of the Victim who transcends the Wheel. *Water* brings understanding, purification, healing.

EARTH The mountain represents the basic bones of Earth, but this most transformative element is also found in the

Tree from which the victim hangs by one of his feet, for the Tree is rooted in Earth, and draws its sustenance directly from the secret UnderWorld. The *Vita* specifically states that the horse 'slipped upon a high rock', and that the victim had 'one of his feet caught in a tree'.

The first image represents the vehicle of energy (Fire) encountering the reflecting or resisting powers of limitation (Earth). The second image is found in the Tarot trump of the Hanged Man, where the figure is hanging by one foot (see description in Chapter 5, and the various pictures in Tarot packs). We should also add to this list that the shock of the fall and sudden suspension from a tree represents a descent through the Elements in terms of spatial order (from the high Air to the low Water and Earth, a flight similar to that of the setting Sun), but the order of encounter is shown in a more subtle manner as in our Figure 12.

Finally the shock of the fall or of hanging traditionally breaks the neck, a physical exaggeration of a spiritual process in which our rigid conceptual views are cracked open, often seeming like death or injury to the assumed personality. In magical or metaphysical practices, the subtle energies of the psychic-body interaction are set into order and amplified by a manipulation of the neck vertebrae, said to be a physical expression of an inner or metaphysical change. This is found in certain wounds or breakages of the neck or collar bone in the Grail legends, and in the worldwide theories on the power centres of the human entity (known in popular Eastern terminology as the *chakras*). *Earth* brings ultimate transformation.

Particular emphasis was given by the ancient Celts to the power of the head; primitive Celts were head hunters; later legends repeatedly assert the magical properties of the head; Merlin, we should remember, wrenches the horns from a stag's head, and uses them to kill a male stereotype false-husband, a reflection of his old self. The Hanged Man has his head in the river, and the vertebrae of the neck connect the head to the body. We might summarise this curious sequence of symbols by stating paradoxically that we think that our bodies have heads, but it is really our heads that have bodies.

The Threefold Death, therefore, shows not only the cycle of Elements in their usual pattern (Air/Fire/Water/Earth; Spring/-Summer/Autumn/Winter; Birth/Adulthood/Maturity/Age; Life/-Light/Love/Law) but a sacrificial or transformative path which cuts across the Wheel, leading to an inner liberation. This is shown in our Figure 12, and moves thus: Air/Fire/Earth/Water; East/South/North/West. The body position of the Hanged Man superimposed upon the Circled Cross will give this configuration, hence the emphasis upon his hanging from a tree by one foot.

The configuration is supported by another traditional position in Celtic folklore and belief, in which a person stands upon one foot, with one hand behind his or her back, and one eye closed (or variants of this theme). This position was used to curse and to see into the Otherworld. It is, if we may allow ourselves the phrase, an upside-down-Hanged-Man, with one foot in the material world instead of upon the Tree of Transformation. It need hardly be added that specific body, hand and foot positions play an important part in yoga, magical workings, and in the general flow of energies through the human entity.

As mentioned in our Chapter 5, the Threefold Death is a very specific magical expression of a theme which is also found in the religious symbolism of the Crucifixion, in addition to pagan sacrificial images which predate the Christian manifestation of the theme. The relationship is a matter of harmonics and metaphysics, but the religious revelation is one of spiritual intuition or, on a lesser scale, of belief. There is no suggestion here that the Threefold Death pre-empt or replaces the Death and Resurrection, merely that such themes are a property of consciousness in all religions through the ages.

APPENDIX VIII
The Lord of the Animals

A little way within the wood thou wilt meet with a road branching off to the right, by which thou must proceed until thou comest to a large sheltered glade with a mound in the centre. And thou wilt see a black man of great stature on top of the mound. He is not smaller in size than two men of this world. He has but one foot and one eye in the middle of his forehead. And he has a club of iron . . . and he is the wood-guardian of that wood. And thou wilt see a thousand wild animals grazing around him . . .

And he took his club in his hand and with it he struck a stag a great blow so that he brayed loudly, and at his braying the animals came together as numerous as the stars in the sky, so that it was difficult for me to find room to stand in the glade amongst them. There were serpents and dragons and divers sort of animals. And he looked upon them, and bade them go and feed; and they bowed their heads and did him homage as vassals to their lord.

The Lady of The Fountain (Mabinogion),
trans. Lady C. Guest.

Bibliographical notes

General bibliographical note: *The Quest For Merlin*, Tolstoy, N., Hamish Hamilton, London, 1985, contains a remarkable historical theory relating to Merlin, and provides a detailed set of research references.

INTRODUCTION

1 *The History of the British Kings: Historia Regum Britanniae* (includes *The Prophecies*), translated Giles, J.A., 1844, London; Thorpe, L., 1966, Harmondsworth. *The Life of Merlin: Vita Merlini*, translated Parry, J.J., 1925, Urbana (University of Illinois), and Clarke, B., 1973, Cardiff. Thorpe, Parry and Clarke include essential notes and commentaries for study of the texts.
2 *The Prophetic Vision of Merlin*, Stewart, R.J., 1986, London. The companion volume to the present book.
3 Sources for the material of the *Vita* include both Celtic and classical literature and traditions, plus oriental fragments. See Parry and Clarke for detailed references.
4 Gerald of Wales: *The Journey through Wales/Description of Wales*, translated Thorpe, L., 1978, Harmondsworth.
5 *The UnderWorld Initiation*, Stewart, R.J., 1985, Wellingborough. See also 2 above.
6 See Appendix I: *Images*; and Chapter 15, note 30.
7 *The Quest of The Holy Grail*, translated Matarasso, P., 1969, Harmondsworth. *The Grail, Quest for the Eternal*, Matthews, J., 1981, London. *At the Table of the Grail*, Matthews, J. (editor), 1984, London.
8 *The Mabinogion*, translated Gantz, J., 1976, Harmondsworth. *Pagan Celtic Britain*, Ross, A., 1974, London. See also Appendix III: *Preiddeu Annwm*.
9 See 2 above.
10 See Appendix II: *People*.
11 See Appendix I: *Images*.

12 *Prelude to Chemistry*, Read, J., 1939/1961, London. *Psychology and Alchemy*, Jung, C.G., 1953, London.
13 *Music, Mysticism and Magic*, Godwin, J., 1986, London.
14 *The White Goddess*, Graves, R., 1961, London. *Hamlet's Mill*, Santillana, G. and von Dechend, H., 1977, Boston.
15 *The Western Way* (Vols. 1 & 2), Matthews, J. and C., London 1985/6.

1 THE OUTER STRUCTURE AND INNER NATURE OF THE *VITA MERLINI*

1 *The Prophetic Vision of Merlin.*
2 See Appendices for examples of related tales or poems, and Chapter 15 for a synthesis of the images.
3 Chapter 5.
4 Chapter 10.
5 *The Druids*, Piggot. S., 1974, Harmondsworth.
6 See Appendix II: *People*: Merlin.
7 *Shamanism: Archaic techniques of ecstacy*, Eliade, M., 1964, New York.
8 The thesis is followed in detail in the commentary on the individual sections of the *Vita*.

2 MERLIN AND MADNESS/THE BATTLE LAMENT

1 'Citharmque sonate.' In an early Welsh context this instrument would have been the *crwth*, a type of bowed lyre or proto-violin. *Relics of the Welsh Bards*, Jones, E., 1784, London (reprinted 1985).
2 Chapter 10. See also Appendix IV: *Creation Poems*.
3 See Appendix V for short summaries of the *Lailoken* and *Suibhne* tales.
4 Chapter 6.
5 *Pagan Celtic Britain*, Ross., 1974, London, Chapter 3.
6 Chapter 14; the theme develops slowly throughout the *Vita*.

3 THE WINTER LAMENT

1 *The Apple Tree* is a recurring image in Celtic poetry.
2 As note 1 for Merlin addressing a pig. See also *The UnderWorld*

Initiation, Stewart, R.J., 1985, Wellingborough, Chapter 6, for a discussion of magical totem beasts.

3 The Wolf is repeatedly associated with CERNUNNOS in early Celtic carvings and emblems. The relationship between the Stag-god and the Wolf is shown in detail in *Pagan Celtic Britain*, Ross, A., 1974, London.

4 *Prelude to Chemistry*, Read, J., 1939/1961, London; *Athanasius Kircher* and *Robert Fludd*, Godwin, J., 1979, London. All show striking examples of such landscapes and images in later symbolism.

5 *Celtic Heritage*, Alwyn and Brinley Rees, 1961, London.

4 THE QUESTION OF THE FOUR SEASONS/LAMENT FOR GUENDOLOENA

1 See Appendix II: *People*.
2 Chapter 10.
3 *Medieval Music, the Sixth Liberal Art*, Hughes, A., 1980, London: a detailed survey of source books and musical studies. *Music and the Elemental Psyche*, Stewart, R.J., 1986, Wellingborough.
4 *The Greek Myths*, Graves, R., 1958, London.
5 See Appendix VI: *The Flower Maiden*.
6 Chapter 5.
7 *Foundations of Tibetan Mysticism*, Govinda, A., 1969, London. *The Rose Cross and The Goddess*, Knight, G., 1985, Wellingborough. *The Cult of The Black Virgin*, Begg, E., 1985, London.

5 MERLIN'S FIRST RETURN/THE THREEFOLD DEATH

1 Wayland is the Titanic smith of Western traditions; maker of magical artifacts. Such smith figures appear throughout world mythology.
2 Compare to chained figure in '*Lord Bateman*', discussed in *The UnderWorld Initiation*, Stewart, R.J., 1985, Wellingborough.
3 See discussion of 'Porter' image, ibid.
4 See Appendix II: *People*: Merlin.
5 *Where is Saint George?* (pagan imagery in folksong), Stewart, R.J., 1977, Bradford on Avon. *Folklore in the English and Scottish Ballads*, Wimberley, L.C., 1959, New York. Ballads discussed in Stewart, 1985, op. cit.

6   Clarke traces the motif to a widespread Indo-European folk tale. (See Introduction, note 1.)

7   Appendix V: *Lailoken and Suibhne*.

8   Chapter 14.

9   *Padstow's Obby Oss*, Rawė, D.R., 1971, Padstow. *Sword Dance and Drama*, Alford, V., 1962, London. *A Harvest of Festivals*, Green, M., 1980, London.

10 *The Prophetic Vision of Merlin*, Stewart, R.J., 1986, London.

11 Chapter 6. Also 'Lord Bateman', Stewart, 1985, op. cit.

12 The approximate date of composition of the *Vita Merlini* is 1150. Discussed in Parry and Clarke (see Introduction, note 1).

13 Celtic religious symbolism is analysed in *Pagan Celtic Britain*, Ross, A., 1974, London, and in *Celtic Heritage*, Rees, A. and B., 1961, London.

14 See Appendix I: *Images*.

15 *Celtic Mysteries*, Sharkey, J., 1975, London. *Celtic Mythology*, MacCana, P., 1975, London. (See also 13 above.)

16 *The Stars in Our Heavens*, Lum, P., London; *Star Names, Their Lore and Meaning*, Allen, Richard Hinckley, New York.

17 Stewart, 1986, op. cit.

18 Chapter 14.

6   MERLIN AND GUENDOLOENA/FIRST STAR-LORE/LORD OF THE ANIMALS

1   *The Golden Bough*, Frazer, J.G., 1907-15, London; see also Introduction, note 14.

2   *The Prophetic Vision of Merlin*, Stewart, R.J., 1986, London.

3   'Lord Bateman', *The UnderWorld Initiation*, Stewart, R.J., 1985, Wellingborough. Also Matthew 22, 3/8/10; Luke 12, 36; Revelation 18, 23; 21, 2/9; 22, 17.

4   Chapter 5.

5   Chapter 9.

6   See Appendix VIII: *The Lord of The Animals*.

7   Chapter 12.

8   See Appendix VI: *The Flower Maiden*.

9   See Chapter 5, note 5.

10 Taliesin in Celtic tradition, Moses in the Old Testament. *The Mabinogion (Taliesin)*, Guest, C., 1904, London.

7 MERLIN'S SECOND RETURN

1 Chapter 8; Matthews, 1981 (Introduction, note 7); Clarke (Introduction, note 1) for examples.
2 *The Prophetic Vision of Merlin*, Stewart, R.J., 1986, London.

8 MERLIN'S OBSERVATORY

1 See Chapter 7, note. 1.
2 *The Legendary History of Britain*, Tatlock, J.S.P., 1950, Berkeley; and see Introduction, note 1.
3 *The Stars and the Stones*, Brennan, M., 1983, London. *The Stone Circles of The British Isles*, Burl, A., 1976, London. *Megalithic Sites in Britain*, Thom, A., 1967, Oxford.
4 See note 2 above.
5 *The Waters of the Gap*, Stewart, R.J., 1981, Bath.
6 *The Mystic Spiral*, Purce, J., 1974, London; *The Stars in Our Heavens*, Lum P., London; *The Round Art*, Mann, A.T., 1979, London; *Star Names, Their Lore and Meaning*, Allen, R.H., New York.
7 It seems unlikely, though, that medieval astrologers employed such minute divisions as those implied in the number seventy. If there is any actual value to the number seventy it might stem from an Eastern source through Arabic cultural transmission. The matter will always be open to argument as it derives from a fusion of traditions.
8 Matthews, 1981, discusses a star-temple in seventh-century Persia (see Introduction, note 7).

9 MERLIN'S PROPHETIC HISTORY/LAMENT FOR RHYDDERCH

1 See *The Life of Merlin: Vita Merlini*, Clarke, B., 1973, Cardiff, for text.
2 See Introduction, note 1.
3 *The Prophetic Vision of Merlin*, Stewart, R.J., 1986, London.
4 Taliesin has been at the school of Gildas the Wise, in Brittany. This historical image is reflective of a Celtic tradition, in which magical or esoteric wisdom is always learned in a school 'over the water' or a 'foreign school'; the school is an allegory for Otherworld instruction. Significantly, Taliesin (Chapter 10) comes up with a mixture of mythical and contemporary natural history or cosomology.

10   THE CREATION OF THE WORLD

1   Classical and derivative medieval sources available to Geoffrey included Solinus, Isidore, and Bede. For a full discussion see Clarke, B., *The Life of Merlin: Vita Merlini*, 1973, Cardiff.
2   Very little hard proof can be offered of 'Druidic' philosophy, but the imagery of late Celtic poems and tales implies an older system of interrelated worlds and dimensions that is never entirely attributable to classical sources. The same argument applies to Geoffrey's mixture of classical and Celtic material in his book.
3   Chapter 4.
4   See Chapter 5, note 5.
5   See Parry and Clarke (Introduction, note 1). A similar vision is found in the *Republic*, Plato; *The Myth of Er*.
6   See Chapter 8, note 5; Introduction, note 5.
7   Appendix III: *Prieddeu Annwm*.
8   These attributes are shared by King Bladud, who is confirmed by archeology with regard to the worship site of Sulis-Minerva and associated carvings (Chapter 8, note 5). If there were no such confirmation the shared attributes might be merely stylish copying of an imaginative theme.
9   *The Prophetic Vision of Merlin*, Stewart, R.J., 1986, London.
10 Chapter 11.
11 Clarke, op. cit.
12 See Appendix II: *People*.

11   MERLIN REMEMBERS/THE THREE FACES OF MERLIN

1   *The History of the Kings of Britain*, Chapter 6-8. See Introduction, notes 1, 2 and 3; Chapter 8, note 2. A full translation of Merlin's 'memoirs' is found in *The Life of Merlin: Vita Merlini*, Clarke, B., 1973, Cardiff.
2   *The Prophetic Vision of Merlin*, Stewart, R.J., 1986, London.

12   THE HEALING FOUNTAIN/MERLIN'S PRAYER/MERLIN'S GREAT AGE

1   Ross, 1974 (Introduction, note 8); Rees, 1961 (Chapter 3, note 5).

2 *Folklore of the Scottish Highlands*, Ross, A., 1976, London.
3 Both knowledge of Ancients and future vision are major elements of *The Prophecies*. See *The Prophetic Vision of Merlin*, Stewart, R.J., 1986, London.
4 Chapter 14.
5 'On one side of the river he saw a flock of white sheep, and on the other a flock of black sheep. And whenever one of the white sheep bleated, one of the black sheep would cross over and become white; and when one of the black sheep bleated, one of the white sheep would cross over and become black. And he saw a tall tree by the side of the river, one half of which was flames from the root to the top, and the other half was green and in full leaf.' *Peredur*, translated by Lady C. Guest.
6 Stewart, op. cit.
7 In *Kilhwch and Olwen (Mabinogion)* a sequence of beasts leads back in time until certain answers are granted, each beast being older than the previous one. One such is the *Stag of Redynvre* who is older than an ancient withered oak tree. Merlin's own connections with a stag and an aged oak tree are clearly part of this myth of the Oldest Creature, either attached to Merlin via oral traditions, or in the form of a magical sequence in which the seer becomes the totem beast himself as an aspect of imaginative power. There is no suggestion that Merlin or the sequence in Kilhwch and Olwen are literary derivatives of one another, but that they share a primal myth which underpins them both.

13   A CATALOGUE OF BIRDS

1 Graves, 1961, (Introduction, note 14) gives a lengthy and detailed discussion of the magical/alphabetic concepts of classical and Celtic cultures, in which the role of the crane features.
2 *The Prophetic Vision of Merlin*, Stewart, R.J., 1986, London.
3 *The White Goddess*, Graves, R., 1961, London; *Hamlet's Mill*, Santillana, G., and von Dechend, H., 1977, Boston; *The Golden Bough*, Frazer, J.G., 1907-15, London.

14   THE POISONED APPLES/THE PROPHECY OF GANIEDA

1 *The UnderWorld Initiation*, Stewart, R.J., 1985, Wellingborough.
2 Thomas Rhymer lived in the thirteenth century, and produced a number of Scottish vernacular prophecies related in many ways to those of Merlin.

3 *The Political Prophecy in England*, Taylor, R.T., 1911, Columbia University.

15 SYNTHESIS: MERLIN, MABON, AND THE RIDDLE OF THREE, FOUR, SIX

1 *Dictionary of Historical Slang*, Partridge, E., Harmondsworth, 1972. The symbolic correlation between 'head' and 'nut' is an important meditational, psychological or magical matter, as the 'head' is traditionally the locus of heightened awareness in metaphysics, while nuts are the seed of wisdom in Celtic tradition. As is often the case, popular slang makes the imaginative connection that was once part of a primal initiatory or magical flow of consciousness.

2 See Introduction, note 8.

3 *Sword Dance and Drama*, Alford, V., 1962, London.

4 *The UnderWorld Initiation*, Stewart, R.J., 1985, Wellingborough.

5 *Trioedd ynys Prydein* (Welsh Triads), ed. Bromwich, R., Cardiff, 1961; see also Introduction, note 8, and Chapter 3, note 5.

6 See Introduction, note 8; Chapter 6, note 10.

7 *Mabon and the Mysteries of Britain*, Matthews, C., London, forthcoming.

8 *The Waters of the Gap*, Stewart, R.J., 1981, Bath.

9 See Introduction, note 8.

10 Stewart, 1985, op. cit.

11 *Mabinogion*, 'Culhwch and Olwen', (various translations).

12 *The Prophetic Vision of Merlin*, Stewart, R.J., 1986, London.

13 It is significant that a number of supernatural beings in Celtic legend have names that identify them with Summer, and that the spirit realm, associated with shadow so frequently, may have once been known as a land of brightness. There is perhaps a faint echo here that it is our human world which is the land of shadow, the realm of ignorance and confusion. Arthur is taken to the Otherworld 'Fortunate Isle' in the *Vita* to be cured of a wound gained through his loss of kingship in the human world.

14 See Chapter 10 for the role of Taliesin; Appendix II: *People* for descriptions of various personae.

15 Chapter 10

16 Appendix II: *People*; Chapter 10.

17 Appendix III: *Preiddeu Annwm*.

18 Stewart, 1986, op. cit.

19 Appendix VI: *The Flower Maiden*; *Mabinogion*, Blodeuedd in 'Math, Son of Mathonwy'.

20 'Culhwch and Olwen', *Mabinogion*.

21 As note 20 above; 'Branwen Daughter of Llyr', *Mabinogion*.

22 'Pwyll Lord of Dyved', *Mabinogion*.

23 As note 22 above; the theme appears in other Mabinogi also.

24 Regenerative themes run through the various Mabinogi.

25 'Branwen, Daughter of Llyr', *Mabinogion*.

26 Chapter 5; Appendix VII: *The Threefold Death*; *Celtic Mythology*, MacCana, P., 1975, London; *Myth and Law among the Indo-Europeans*, Puhvel, J., (ed.), 1970, Berkeley.

27 Chapter 5.

28 In 'Culhwch and Olwen' the hero claims the right to have his hair trimmed by King Arthur, who thus discovers him to be a kinsman, his first cousin.

29 Such role-changing dramas form the core of a ritual known in the ancient world, originally connected to actual human sacrifice, but later rationalised or substituted by a symbolic act often claimed as the origin of all theatre. In late Roman culture criminals were 'selected' for the role-change-sacrifice, thus preserving a system that was no longer understood.

30 An early reference is the banning of cards in 1332 by King Leon of Castile. Cards commissioned by Charles VI of France (1392) are still preserved in the Bibliothèque Nationale; these are the origin of many later Tarot images. By the fifteenth and sixteenth centuries *Tarrochi* packs of over one hundred cards were known as images for education in addition to their use in games of chance. The Tarot known as the 'traditional' Marseilles pack is as late as the eighteenth century.

31 Stewart, 1986, op. cit.

32 *Summa Secunda Secundae Quest*; clxxx, Art vi vid, Appendix Latine.

33 'Math, Son of Mathonwy', *Mabinogion*, in which Arianrhod gives birth; *History of The British Kings* (Book V, Ch. XVII), in which Merlin has an accusing companion or twin; *The Rosicrucians, their Rites and Mysteries*, Jennings, H., 1887, London.

34 Chapter 5; Appendix VII: *The Threefold Death*.

35 *The Hymn of Jesus* (from *The Leucian Acts*), trans. Mead, G.R.S.

Index